KU-312-371

Negotiating Health Care

The Social Context
of Chronic Illness

SALLY E. THORNE

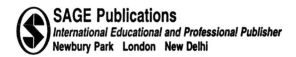
SAGE Publications
International Educational and Professional Publisher
Newbury Park   London   New Delhi

Copyright © 1993 by Sage Publications, Inc.

All rights reserved. No part of this book may be reproduced or utilized in any form or by any means, electronic or mechanical, including photocopying, recording, or by any information storage and retrieval system, without permission in writing from the publisher.

For information address:

SAGE Publications, Inc.
2455 Teller Road
Newbury Park, California 91320

SAGE Publications Ltd.
6 Bonhill Street
London EC2A 4PU
United Kingdom

SAGE Publications India Pvt. Ltd.
M-32 Market
Greater Kailash I
New Delhi 110 048 India

Printed in the United States of America

Library of Congress Cataloging-in-Publication Data

Thorne, Sally E. (Sally Elizabeth), 1951-
    Negotiating health care: the social context of chronic illness /
Sally E. Thorne.
        p.   cm.
    Includes bibliographical references and index.
    ISBN 0-8039-4917-0 (cl).—ISBN 0-8039-4918-9
    1. Chronic diseases—Social aspects.   2. Chronic diseases—
Psychological aspects.   3. Chronically ill—Public opinion.
4. Chronically ill—Attitudes.   5. Chronically ill—Medical care—
Public opinion.   6. Medical personnel and patient.   I. Title.
    [DNLM: 1. Chronic Disease.   2. Delivery of Health Care.
3. Negotiating.   4. Professional—Patient Relations.   WT 30 T511n
1993]
RA644.5.T49   1993
362.1—dc20   92-48444
                                                                                      CIP

94 95 96   10 9 8 7 6 5 4 3 2

Sage Production Editor: Judith L. Hunter

Accession no.
00993651

WITHDRAWN

16.95

WT 30 THO

362.19 THO

**This book is to be returned on or before
the last date stamped below.**

13 DEC 1995

- 5 APR 2000

1

Negotiating
Health Care

Contents

Acknowledgments

When a book represents the fruits of your life work to date, acknowledging all who made a significant contribution poses a preposterous challenge. I would have to dig quite deeply into my own past to name all who encouraged my academic and professional development. More recently, I have benefitted from an army of teachers, colleagues, and co-conspirators in my attempts to learn about the experience of chronic illness and to make some sense of it within the strange social world we all inhabit. I have been blessed by knowing inspirational people all of my life, and I consider the women and men in my own social and professional world as the central source of anything that I have to offer here. I hope that they know how deeply I feel their influence. Having declared that my acknowledgments will only scratch the surface of the list deserving recognition, I will name a few whose contributions to this project were distinctive and significant. I am indebted to my co-investigator in the original health care relationships project, Carole Robinson, to the team involved in that research, including Mary Adlersberg, Elizabeth Ann Armstrong, Marie Bennett, and Shelley Canning, and to the University of British Columbia School of Nursing, where the ideas were conceived and nurtured. One of the great privileges within my career has been the opportunity, through the Union Institute for Advanced Studies, to compile a unique panel of experts to guide and support me through the intricacies of the research that led to this book. These wonderful people are: Marci Catanzaro, Barbara Dobbie, Jan Kido, Hal Kirshbaum, Juliene Lipson, and Penny MacElveen-Hoehn. Another group of people, who provided suppport through the process of manuscript preparation, revision, and (especially) reduction, consisted of Jane Ellis, Marjorie Sinel, Dale Walker, and the wonderful crew at Sage Publications, Inc., including Judy Hunter, Julie Marshall, and Christine Smedley. Next, I must acknowledge the sustained support of a colorful and exceptional family and friendship network, most especially my daughter, Leah. Finally, I would like to thank the many women, men, and children with chronic illness or with a chronically ill loved one who permitted their very private lives to be made public because they were committed to making a difference. The passion and integrity in their stories has challenged me to understand the world quite differently from when I first began. I hope that this book does some justice to their realities and to the social context into which their accounts permit us a glimmer of understanding.

Preface

Health care in modern industrialized nations is in desperate trouble. Once cherished as the most prestigious and respected of professions, medicine is now the focus of extensive litigation and general public criticism. The proliferation of medical technology, once proclaimed as testimony to the supremacy of democracy and a free market economy, has transformed Western biomedical care from a humanitarian social service into a profitable corporate enterprise. Costs have skyrocketed, exhausting funds needed to support other sectors of the public domain. Dissatisfaction among health care professionals, health care workers, and health care consumers is epidemic in proportion.

The literature documenting and analyzing the current health care crisis is voluminous. It contains the critical wisdom of philosophy, sociology, psychology, anthropology, the health sciences, and numerous other disciplines. This book adds another voice to those that have already been heard on the subject. It represents one nurse researcher's interpretation of the perspective of an underrepresented stakeholder in the debate, that of the chronically ill.

The chronically ill, by far the largest health care consumer population in urban industrialized nations, have a uniquely vested interest in the health of the health care system. They observe it and participate in it over extended periods of time, seeking from it whatever comfort and aid is available, coming into contact with a range of individual providers and services. Because their circumstances force them into intimate contact with the health care system in its various manifestations, they develop their own analysis of its character and its peculiarities. Further, they tend to become highly frustrated with, and insightful about, its very real limitations.

A great deal has been written about chronic illness in our society. Psychologists have considered its personality correlates, sociologists have interpreted its social implications, economists have determined its social cost, anthropologists have explored its cultural shaping, and analysts with a philosophical bent have investigated its subjective meaning to those afflicted. While each of these approaches offers an original perspective of the phenomenon, each is limited by the angle of its scope and the precision of its focus. Just as chronic illness experience cannot be understood by merely concentrating on the molecular change that characterizes a chronic disease, the subjective experience of chronic illness cannot be captured in isolation from the social and institutional contexts in which it occurs. One such context, and a profoundly important one, is the dysfunctional health care system within which the chronically ill are forced to negotiate for the supports and services essential to a decent quality of life.

This book, therefore, has a twofold purpose. The first is to chronicle the complexity of chronic illness experience in our modern world through a description of what it is like to be chronically ill. The second is to apply this account of the chronic illness experience toward an understanding of the flaws in modern health care organization and ideology.

It is evident that the dialectic between chronic illness experience and the larger social context in which it occurs cannot be reduced to straightforward analytic categories or to a neat, linear association. Like all such complex social relationships, this one is untidy, confusing, and at times even contradictory; and although it defeats simplistic explanation, I believe it worthy of serious inquiry. Practical knowledge of the chronic illness experience and its context are unlikely to be gleaned from a single clever insight, metaphor, or conceptual framework offered by this or any other author. Rather, I encourage the reader to engage in the intense acts of "making sense" of the phenomenon, empathizing with it, and carefully judging its truth value. From this foundation, it is my hope that a critical understanding of human and social experience in health care will emerge. I therefore offer the reader not the final answer to any of the very profound and penetrating questions facing health care reform, but rather an alternative perspective from which to ponder the underlying meaning of questions that all of us must eventually ask.

ONE

Background to the
Chronic Illness Experience

At the age of 45, David Rabin was Director of Endocrinology at the Vanderbilt Medical Center. His research in the fields of metabolism and reproduction was flourishing. He and his wife travelled extensively and enjoyed an active social life until Dr. Rabin began to experience the first signs of Amyotrophic Lateral Sclerosis (ALS, commonly known as Lou Gehrig's disease), a chronic progressive neurologic condition that eventually paralyzed him completely. While Dr. Rabin was well aware that there was no known cure for this disease, he was totally unprepared for how profoundly it would affect his remaining productive years. Where they had once treated him as an esteemed peer, his colleagues now took pains to avoid him. Physician friends immediately broke off all communication. His wife was treated as a premature widow by friends she encountered socially. In short, he was considered an outcast.

The Rabins reckoned that if this had happened to them in their enlightened social network, then it must also happen to others. They published an article in a prestigious medical journal documenting the reaction of fellow physicians to their illness. The response was overwhelming. Chronically ill physicians from all over the world expressed pain, anguish, and despair in a flood of letters and phone calls. Thus the Rabins came to appreciate that chronic illness is a social disease in the context of modern medical ideology (Rabin & Rabin, 1985).

The experience of the Rabins is disturbing, not because it reveals an aberration, but because it is so very predictable. It illustrates the degree to which the social world and a specific disease process interact to create an illness experience for those involved. Further, it shows us how far apart are the objective medical view of a disease and the subjective personal experience. An ironic note to Dr. Rabin's story was that he had earlier rejected a career in clinical neurology because he reasoned that the diagnostic problems were mere academic exercises in the absence of definitive therapeutics (Rabin, Rabin, & Rabin, 1985). If you can't cure the problem, what then is the point?

The point of studying chronic illness is much larger than simply the hope of curing chronic disease. It has to do with the very essence of human aspirations and meanings. People do not become less human, less interesting, or less deserving just because they have unresolvable or disabling conditions. Rather, they continue to learn, to adapt, and to live their lives as well as they can manage. In other words, they seek a state of health that represents their best effort within the specific challenges of their disease. And helping people to achieve this health is, after all, what the health care system is supposed to be about.

CHRONIC ILLNESS EXPERIENCE

What we know about chronic illness experience is limited and fragmented. Until quite recently, it was difficult to justify doing research on a vague and nonspecific issue such as "chronic illness." Instead, scholars were encouraged to study aspects of particular diseases, the idea being to understand each disease as a distinct entity (Rolland, 1988). However, this approach denied the more experiential nature of chronic illness, in that sufferers seem to have much more in common than was previously thought possible (Strauss, Corbin, Fagerhaugh, Glaser, Maines, Suczek, & Wiener, 1984).

The term *chronic* refers to diseases of long duration, in which there may be little change or slow progression. It is the opposite of *acute*, the kind of disease that we acquire and, hopefully, resolve fairly quickly. Despite the cherished myth in our society that chronic diseases are not terribly serious (or are at least not life-threatening), most of us will eventually die of one (Burish & Bradley, 1983). Among chronic diseases there are those that are painful and those that are not, those that will eventually result in death and those that will not influence mortality, those that disfigure or disable and those that influence a person in more subtle and invisible ways (Nordstrom & Lubkin, 1990). The similarity between them is that the problem cannot normally be "fixed" by modern health care methods (Curtin & Lubkin, 1990).

Although the epidemiological picture of chronic illness is difficult to portray accurately (Kasl, 1983), all estimates suggest that chronic illness is the most serious health problem of the latter half of this century (Myers, 1988), affecting about one-third of the population at any time (Lohr, Kamberg, Keeler, Goldberg, Calabro, & Brook, 1987). Further, it is well established that the prevalence of chronic illness is increasing due to factors such as changing life-style trends and the aging of the population (Jekel, 1987; Last, 1987).

Much of our knowledge of the chronic illness experience derives from attempts to understand the psychological and social consequences of being ill over time. Chronic illnesses tend to be long-term, uncertain in course, and disproportionately intrusive on the lives of those who experience them (Strauss et al., 1984). Changes resulting from a chronic illness tend to be cyclical and compound the impact of previous changes (Strauss & Corbin, 1988). Some of the more inevitable problems include intrafamilial stresses, social isolation, frustrations with independence, insults to the self-image, and economic pressures (Curtin & Lubkin, 1990). The chronically ill individual and his or her family may well find these illness-related changes to be far more problematic than the disease itself.

A substantial body of literature is devoted to sorting out why some patients and families seem to adapt successfully to chronic illness and why others do not (Diamond, 1983). Traditionally, studies of adaptation have attempted to correlate outcomes with mental attributes of the patient and somatic properties of the disease (Shonz, 1984). An alternative approach has been to document the psychosocial demands illness creates. Various authors have recognized that minimizing the necessary life-style adaptations, gaining control over treatment, managing emotions, and acquiring information are common elements within chronic illness experience (Baron, 1987; Lambert & Lambert, 1987; Larkin, 1987; Salmond, 1987; Tilden & Weinert, 1987).

The literature on coping with chronic illness draws heavily upon theories of adaptation and coping. Moos and Tsu's (1977) typology of common coping skills is considered pioneering work in the study of coping in physical illness. Another substantial body of theory is attributed to Lazarus and colleagues, who articulated the influence of cognitive appraisal in coping responses, concluding that there are no inherently adaptive or maladaptive coping strategies (Cohen & Lazarus, 1983). The seminal work of Strauss and others in "illness trajectory" extends the traditional idea of coping into an interpretation of long-term patterns in chronic illness experience (Corbin & Strauss, 1988; Strauss, 1981; Strauss, Fagerhaugh, Suczek, & Wiener, 1981; Wiener, Fagerhaugh, Strauss, & Suczek, 1984). According to this perspective, the problems of chronic illness are less a product of the physiological unfolding of the course of disease than of the organization of illness work in conjunction with the illness (Strauss et al., 1984; Strauss & Corbin, 1988).

Another significant focus in the study of chronic illness experience has been in the area of "illness behavior." This approach recognizes that people do not uniformly conclude that they are ill or seek treatment on the basis of similar symptoms or for similar reasons (Morgan, Calnan, & Manning, 1985). It claims that what is defined and recorded as illness is explained better by social than by medical factors (Leventhal, Nerenz, & Straus, 1982; Zola, 1973). The work of Mechanic and others has generated a valuable body of theory on how people interpret and cope with various illness conditions (Alonzo, 1984; Frankel & Nuttall, 1984; Mechanic, 1983, 1986b, 1989). Among the most popular offshoots of the illness behavior work is the "health beliefs model," originally formulated by Rosenstock (1966) and later developed by Becker and colleagues (Becker, 1974; Becker, Haefner, Kasl, Kirscht, Maiman, & Rosenstock, 1977). This psychological learning approach linked motivation, values, and cognitions to health-related behavior. Numerous variables presumed to affect health behavior differences have been subjected to scrutiny through the use of this model (Gallagher, 1988; Mikhail, 1981).

Anthropological inquiries have focused attention on the meaning of illness behavior. Scholars such as Fabrega (1974) have long considered illness to be a cultural construct. Interpretive approaches in this area have brought forth a school of thought characterized by the "explanatory model of illness" (Young, 1982). According to this approach, each culture organizes its ideas about illness according to certain core symbolic elements. Kleinman, the most influential among these theorists, has brought the field full circle by linking the semantic networks people bring to their illness with their systems of medical knowledge (Kleinman, 1980; Kleinman, Eisenberg, & Good, 1978).

A related source of understanding about chronic illness experience emerges from phenomenological descriptions that have begun to appear in the scholarly literature (Brody, 1987; Buchanan, 1989; Kaufman, 1988; Krefting, 1990; Radley, 1989; Ruffing-Rahal, 1985; Scambler & Hopkins, 1986). While each investigation employs a distinct angle of vision, they collectively reinforce the idea that chronic illness experience is embedded in the structural realities and cultural knowledge inherent in the social world of the patient. The notion of "meaning" is a recurrent theme in this body of literature. According to Pellegrino (1982), illness represents an assault on the unity of being, eroding the images we have constructed of ourselves and the world. Because meaning is not automatically ascribed to illness experience in our culture, making meaning becomes an essential element in the way an illness is experienced (Lenihan, 1981). Various authors have attempted to document the kinds of meaning people make of their illnesses (Herzlich & Graham, 1973; Mann, 1982; Stephenson & Murphy, 1986), producing powerful images of the many ways in which physical distress is embedded within our psychosocial metaphors.

Thus, our understanding of chronic illness experience is informed by the contributions of a wide range of disciplines and perspectives. Epidemiologically, we appreciate chronic illness as an experience shared by an increasing proportion of the population. Psychologically, we recognize it as a significant affliction requiring continual adaption and coping. From a social interaction perspective, we know that it radically alters the essential structure of our human relationships. And from the insights of the more philosophically inclined scholars, we begin to recognize the loaded imagery inherent in the idea of becoming and staying ill in our society.

The research to date has provided us with insights about patterns in disease progress and correlates of symptomatic distress. We know, for example, that anxious people feel their pain more strongly, that fear keeps some people from seeking help, and that uncertainty about the prognosis of disease is usually more upsetting than is knowledge of a certain outcome. However, as any clinician or patient knows, individual experiences are rather more unique and mysterious than statistical norms suggest. Thus, there is a resurgence of enthusiasm for methods of understanding illness experience that account for its inherent subjectivity (Calnan, 1987).

Because it is complex and multifaceted, the subjective experience of chronic illness is very difficult to study. One approach is to ask people what they think, to have them articulate their experience, and to record it as faithfully as possible. However, with the exception of poets and artists, few people are skilled at expressing their subjective experience so that other people can truly understand. Most of us are trapped in a limited vocabulary, stopped short when it comes to conveying abstractions, and completely mute with regard to the deepest and darkest elements in our subconscious minds. A skilled interviewer can bring forth more than what might otherwise be available; however, the introduction of another person into the interaction raises the specter of bias, misinterpretation and distortion of the message in unpredictable ways (Armstrong, 1984).

Another complication in studying subjective experience is that not all of what affects us will ever be accessible to consciousness. Anthropological and sociological inquiry has convincingly revealed that we all understand the world according to the dictates of our socialization and culture. Much of what we know is tacit knowledge in that we rely on it, but could probably never articulate it. Such knowledge guides our behavior and emotions in socially acceptable ways and shapes the way we believe our world ought to be organized. The individual is often a poor source for such information; instead, one needs to explore shared elements in the experience of many people in order to begin identifying patterns that might explain common subjective features.

Subjective explorations to this point have revealed that people experience chronic illness in the context of their family and immediate social universe (Gilliss, Rose, Hallburg, & Martinson, 1989; Morse & Johnson, 1991; Rolland, 1987). When one member of a family is ill, the whole family is disrupted, and this disruption may well be the most meaningful element in the illness experience for all concerned (Leahey & Wright, 1987). We also know that our society has specific expectations for the behavior of an ill person. Instead of complete submission to events that befall him or her, the ill person is expected to cope, to figure out how to manage the stresses and strains brought on by the illness in ways that maintain as normal a life as possible (Tagliacozzo & Mauksch, 1979).

These findings make it clear that the subjective experience of living with a chronic disease is far more complex than simply bearing pain, feeling fatigued, or living with the physical symptoms that the disease or its treatment might bring on (Conrad, 1990; Gerhardt, 1990). Rather, it is an entity constructed by the many forces at play in the interaction between ourselves and our social worlds (Bury, 1991). Indeed, the chronic illness experience is a highly charged social phenomenon.

SOCIAL IMPLICATIONS OF CHRONIC ILLNESS

As was evident in the account of Rabin's transition from physician to pariah, chronic illness can represent a radical departure from the social world of the robust and able-bodied. When a person is treated differently, he or she begins to feel different in response. Thus, a person and his or her social world engage in an intense dialectic in which the experience of any given chronic illness is shaped.

Sociologists who have studied the fascinating nature of this interaction offer various theories about how and why this dialectic operates. The social world discredits those with various health differences, rendering them incompetent and invalid if not invisible. Many of the chronic illnesses carry with them the potential of stigma, the metaphoric imagery that bestows certain symbolic meanings on certain disease conditions. Thus, the chronically ill may be variously considered unclean, weak-willed, contagious, defective, or immoral (Brody, 1987).

Sick role theory, as articulated by Parsons (1951, 1979) and developed by his successors, expresses the relationship of sick people to their society in terms of the roles and obligations expected of patients and experts. Although some have argued that sick role theory is less applicable to chronic illness than to acute illness (Meleis, 1988), many believe that the sickness contract embedded in our social structure convincingly explains many of the confusing messages that the chronically ill receive about how they ought to conduct their lives (Alexander, 1982; Cockerham, 1986; Lubkin, 1990b).

While everyone within the social universe of any chronically ill person has the potential to create havoc, perhaps none are so excruciatingly influential upon the whole experience as are the health care professionals on whom the patient becomes reliant (Arney & Bergen, 1984). According to common social logic, health care professionals are expected to be moral leaders in equity, dignity, and justice (Gething, 1992). As a result of this, the relationships between patients and providers have traditionally been viewed with mere curiosity and not consternation. The study of health care relationships has been fragmented and disjointed, in part because scholars have based their inquiries on a wide range of mutually incompatible theoretical models (Hahn, Feiner, & Bellin, 1988; Mizrahi, 1986; Pendleton, 1983). Much of the research addresses the "clinical encounter" as a microcosm of the broader issues involved in health care relationships. Such studies have effectively documented predictable miscommunication patterns, incompatible expectations, and the influence of doctor-patient communications on clinical decision making (Bochner, 1983; Fisher, 1984; Marshall, 1988; Mishler, 1984; Paget, 1983; Robinson & Whitfield, 1988; West, 1984).

Another branch of the research has explored the attitudes of health care professionals toward their patients for insight about endemic problems in health care relationships. These studies reveal that health care professionals are often insensitive to the impact of their discourse upon patients (Bourhis, Roth, & MacQueen, 1989), distrustful of the involvement of family members (Yoder & Jones, 1982), and increasingly disinclined toward cooperative models of health care (Sparr, Gordon, Hickam, & Girard, 1988). Correspondingly, studies of how patients perceive medical encounters further document the extent of the problem. Several researchers have concluded that dissatisfaction with such encounters is widespread (Lau, Williams, Williams, Ware, & Brook, 1982) and that it has a detrimental effect on both the psychological and the medical effectiveness of the consultation (Charmaz, 1983; Fitzpatrick, Hopkins, & Harvard-Watts, 1983; Jaspars, King, & Pendleton, 1983). Such dissatisfaction is strongly linked to issues of communication between health care providers and patients (Buller & Buller, 1987; Like & Zyanski, 1987).

A number of controversies flourish in the theoretical literature on health care relationships. Among these are the degree to which patients want input into their care (Sherlock, 1986), and the type of health care relationship that would best meet their needs (Pellegrino & Thomasma, 1988; Rosenstein, 1986). Another hotly debated issue is the role expectations of patients and physicians (Amundsen & Ferngren, 1983). According to Preston (1986), medicine's fundamental deception is the idea that doctors have special healing powers. This culturally embedded notion has been described as the source of numerous systematic errors in medical practice in that it contributes to the willingness of patients to submit to untold indignities, and to the reluctance of physicians to relinquish divine rule. The role of the patient also attracts considerable attention. While sickness confers freedom from the usual role expectations, it requires one to take socially prescribed measures to try to get well (Lambert & Lambert, 1985). Indeed, several researchers have documented the risks patients believe they face if they fail to conform to these social expectations (Appelbaum & Roth, 1983; Lorber, 1979; Tagliacozzo & Mauksch, 1979; Taylor, 1970).

As Illich (1975) and Anderson and Helm (1979) have so aptly pointed out, health care relationships seem to be inherently conflictual social processes. As a society, we labor under the illusion of benevolent medical relationships, whereas doctors and their patients are most often locked in an intense semi-adversarial union (Todd, 1989). This seems to be especially true in the case of chronic illnesses (Gallagher, 1988; Illich, 1975; Tagliacozzo & Mauksch, 1979). Therefore, those most in need of effective health care relationships over time have the least success in sustaining them (Calnan, 1984; Thorne & Robinson, 1988a).

Thus, the literature provides ample evidence that social (and especially health care) interaction features powerfully in the lived experience of chronic illness. It considers the social structure of chronic illness to be an intricately constructed dialectic dependent on culturally embedded assumptions and values governing the behaviors and actions of all of the players involved.

STRUCTURAL IMPLICATIONS OF CHRONIC ILLNESS

Chronic illness care is typically provided by professionals educated toward acute curative models, and in structures designed to provide emergency and highly technological services (Margolese, 1987; Strauss, 1990). The way health care is organized in modern industrialized nations features the most expensive professionals as primary decision makers, a preference for the most technologically oriented services available, and an enthusiasm for discovering exotic curative procedures. Decisions about health care structure, organization, and resource allocation have been dominated by cultural assumptions of the medical profession (McKinlay & Stoeckle, 1988; Navarro, 1986; O'Neill, 1986; Zola, 1981).

This system of health care is in a state of crisis. No Western nation can afford to continue augmenting health care expenditures in the pattern that has characterized recent decades (Callahan, 1992; DeVries, 1988; Evans, 1991; McLennan & Meyer, 1989; Mechanic, 1989). It has become difficult to justify funding increases in health care while populations are becoming sicker and the link between health care spending and the health of populations is becoming weaker (McKeown, 1979; McKinlay & McKinlay, 1987; McKinlay, McKinlay, Jennings, & Grant, 1983). In addition, Western societies have been remarkably reluctant to tackle the ethical dilemmas incited by the "spare no expense" philosophy within medical science. Because expensive procedures threaten to cripple the economy if allowed to proliferate unchecked (Simmons & Marine, 1984), no nation can make them available unconditionally. However, the idea of rationing is so culturally unacceptable (and politically dangerous) in many democratic nations that the profound social issues are left unresolved (Besharov & Silver, 1989; Daniels, 1985). Thus, according to many social planners, we are on the brink of catastrophic change in our understanding of health care organization and delivery (Califano, 1986; Fox, 1986; Inlander, Levin, & Wiener, 1988; McKeown, 1988).

The health care system is made up of numerous professional bodies, each with its own piece of the action to defend, an increasingly large administrative sector and, of course, private industry (which is always heavily involved whether or not health care is nationalized) (Marmor & Dunham, 1983). Although most of our health problems are chronic in nature, we tend to consider our health care system as our insurance against death and make decisions about it accordingly. The structure and function of the system we have created is thus far better suited to the demands of acute illness than it is to the needs of the chronically ill (Meyerson & Herman, 1987; Strauss & Corbin, 1988; Williams, 1991).

In order to effect any major remedy to the health care crisis, the basic philosophies of individual culpability, curative medicine, and biological solutions must be reconsidered (Carlson, 1975). By monopolizing authority over all manner of human conditions, the medical profession has systematically created the impression that solutions to health problems lie in medical innovations (Taylor, 1979). However, according to many health care analysts, the only hope for the present predicament is to emphasize total population systems of health promotion and disease prevention, and to conscientiously address the social, political, and economic problems underlying unhealthy living patterns (Harris, 1989; Hunt, 1988; Rachlis, 1991; Rachlis & Kushner, 1989).

Clearly, the crisis in health care is a serious and complex social problem. Logic tells us that it must have a profound impact on those who are dependent on it for ongoing management of a chronic health condition. However, the nature of that impact has rarely been a focus of scholarly inquiry.

APPROACH TO THE CURRENT RESEARCH

The interaction between the various dimensions of chronic illness experience is rarely an explicit focus of inquiry (Bury, 1991; Herzlich & Pierret, 1985). Those who study individual cases acknowledge that larger social and political decisions play a role; those who interpret epidemiological findings note that they hardly scratch the surface of human experience. However, the dialectic between the grand and the small pictures in chronic illness fails to attract much analysis and scholarship (Strauss & Corbin, 1988). It is too messy to study, its relationships are too complex, and its scope is too immense to provide the focus and direction necessary for investigation that yields any practical value (Pelto & DeWalt, 1985).

Another reason that the macro and micro pictures are so often considered separately is the "culture" of academia, which shapes the territory and methods of each of the relevant disciplines. The norms of each discipline dictate the boundaries and acceptable methodological approaches quite differently (Bennett, 1985). A practice discipline such as nursing, long considered a poor cousin to the pure social and natural sciences, may have a distinct advantage in that it has had to borrow from so many interdisciplinary worldviews. Further, it has sustained a fascination with application because of its practice mandate. Because it deals with large issues, it needs and relies on grand level theories. However, since accounting for application must always reflect the individual level, it demands that these grand theories make sense where actual people are concerned. While this unique challenge may well have delayed nursing's scientific progress, it has provided a fortunate legacy in the adventurous scholarly spirit that permits nurse researchers to step outside their disciplinary boundaries, encourages them to consider the interplay between those large and small pictures, and assures them that the ultimate test will be none other than the usefulness of the ideas in the real world of patients and practitioners.

The value underlying the approach of this book is a conviction that chronic illness experience cannot be fully understood at the physiological, individual, social interpersonal, or structural institutional levels of analysis alone. All will be equally important in creating this abstraction known as the chronic illness experience (Katz, 1987). Further, attempts to understand any of these levels in isolation from the others short-circuits the potential for discovering its meaning to the whole phenomenon. Thus, one cannot fully understand the experience of chronically ill people without understanding what happens in the health care relationships they form and in the experiences they encounter in the larger health care system.

The research upon which this book is based began with a series of qualitative explorations of chronic illness experience, focused increasingly on the societal context in which that experience was shaped (Robinson & Thorne, 1985; Thorne, 1985, 1986, 1988, 1990a, 1990b;

Thorne & Robinson, 1988a, 1988b, 1988c, 1989). Despite efforts to have chronically ill patients and their family members describe their own experiences without interpretation, the accounts were always full of analysis and explanation. As Gubrium might have described them, the people I interviewed were "everyday philosophers" with a stock of systematic resources for "making sense of things" (1988, p. 14). In other words, they made it clear that, if I truly wanted to find out what it was like to be chronically ill, I had better look closely at the system in which these people were immersed.

This challenge led me to the "naturalistic inquiry" that is the subject of this book. For the methodologically inclined reader, a detailed discussion of the design application is provided in the Appendix. The organizational structure of the book reflects a logic validated in the primary and secondary analysis conducted in this research. I understand chronic illness experience to operate at three distinct but interrelated conceptual levels: the individual, the social, and the structural. The three parts of this book follow this pattern, extending the analysis of interaction between these levels as the book progresses.

In relying heavily on the voice of the expert witnesses within the narration of the account, I hope to be able to share with the reader some of the discovery and intuitive understanding I have been privileged to experience over the course of studying chronic illness experience. I invite the reader to approach this book as an abstraction of the voices of those who have experienced a sector of our society, the health care sector, in a way that we may not have, although chances are high that many of us will be among the chronically ill before our lives are through. From the window of their experience, we have the opportunity for a better appreciation of the social and health care universes that we all too often take for granted.

PART ONE

The Individual Experience

Onset and Diagnosis

The chronic illness experience can begin in a variety of ways. Sometimes it originates with almost imperceptible differences in sensation or movement; at other times it emerges in the aftermath of an acute health crisis. Sometimes it is characterized by rapid and frightening changes in the body; at other times it begins with awakening to the realization that familiar symptoms may signal something serious. Some people are born with health problems that will become chronic; others have not yet experienced any bodily changes at all when informed that they are victim to a chronic disease. While there is no single sequence in which onset and diagnosis of chronic illness occur, these events are profoundly important within the chronic illness experience (Hingson, Scotch, Sorenson, & Swazey, 1981; Rolland, 1988).

In this chapter, the interrelated phenomena of illness onset and medical diagnosis will be addressed from the perspective of the ill people involved. A sampling of their stories will illustrate not only the great variety of onset and diagnosis experiences, but also the common patterns that emerge when people seek professional help in trying to understand what is wrong.

THE ONSET OF ILLNESS

No single onset pattern characterizes all chronic illnesses; rather, there is a range that varies from insidious progressive symptom development over a period of years to sudden, acute illness or injury from which full recovery does not occur. Whatever the pattern, the stories of patients and families often begin with an account of illness onset, a recounting of "how it all began."

Some of the informants in this study recalled an acute episode that, for them, marked the beginning of the illness odyssey. For example, one mother remembered the beginning of her child's career with asthma as a sudden wheezing episode that required a 4-day hospitalization. For others, particularly those dealing with progressive, degenerative conditions, the onset of illness was far more difficult to pinpoint. Often, the beginning was marked by the first time that it occurred to them to seek medical assistance for annoying or irritating physical symptoms they had had for some time.

When there was no obvious beginning point, informants searched into their past for some occurrence that might be considered the onset. For example, one man claimed he had not felt well since surgery to remove shrapnel from his stomach during the Second World War. "I mean, I felt workably well, but I never felt good." Other chronically ill individuals recalled being sickly as children, being accident-prone, or having always experienced vague physical symptoms, as one woman's recollections illustrate.

> I am not sure that I wasn't always somebody who wasn't in optimal health. As a teenager, particularly, or as a child, I don't think I ever really had the energy I felt I should have, but nothing was ever identified.

For these chronically ill individuals and their families, then, it seemed important to be able to identify something which signified a beginning point in the experience.

According to these informants, "becoming chronically ill" was a process that included not only the onset of symptoms but also the actual medical diagnosis at some point along the way. For many, the symptoms preceded the diagnosis, sometimes by decades, as one young man's story suggests.

> I can't tell you a day in my life, or a year that it started . . . and I can remember back to the age of 4. I was chronically constipated, and there was something wrong, because I couldn't go to the bathroom when I wanted to, have a bowel movement when it was normal to. So the doctors were pretty unsympathetic. I mean, like I said, I was blamed for it, because I wasn't eating a proper diet and I wasn't going to the bathroom when I was supposed to, stuff like that . . . Intuitively, I knew I was in for something pretty big. Like I knew that there was something else going on and this was part of it. But nobody would listen to me 'cause I was so small.

In his case, his age and the non-specific nature of the symptoms seemed to contribute to the problem of diagnosis. For other patients and families, diagnosis was hampered by what they later recognized as characteristics of the disease itself. One women with scleroderma accounted for her years of illness prior to diagnosis this way.

> It is an insidious disease. It's like a cancer in the way that it spreads internally, and it hits each person differently. That's what makes it difficult to diagnose. There's no blood test that will tell you, there's no X-rays [that] will show, until you have reached the stage where everything has calcified to a point, and the calcium comes out of your skin and your fingers in crystals. And you have to be that far along before a doctor—and it has to be the right doctor, because they're not even trained to think scleroderma.

In other cases, the diagnosis was suggested long before the importance of symptoms had hit home to the patient. One man with Multiple Sclerosis (MS) recalled an event that preceded his acknowledgment of chronic illness onset by several years.

> After awhile, I was called back to [the doctor's] office, and he says, "I've got some news that's not going to be very pleasant." He says, "You've got an illness that's going to really set you on your bottom." And I says, "What are you talking about?" And he says, "Well I'm pretty sure that you've got Multiple Sclerosis." Well, at that time I had never even heard the name and I said, "Multiple what?" and he said, "Multiple Sclerosis." And I said, "Well, what does that do to a person?" He says, "Well, eventually you'll be in a wheelchair." And I said, "You're crazy." And I left him. I never went back to him.

No matter what the chronology of events, the diagnosis itself stood out in the accounts of these informants as a major milestone, a turning point in the process of becoming chronically ill. Whether the implications of chronic illness were appreciated long before, coincident with, or long after the actual medical diagnosis, this event best characterized the experience of entering into chronic illness for these informants. The following discussion of the early chronic illness period will address several distinct aspects of this diagnostic process that featured in the accounts of the patients and families in this study: the diagnostic testing process, the occasion of hearing the diagnosis, the meaning embedded in the diagnosis, and the impact of having received a diagnosis.

THE DIAGNOSTIC TESTING PROCESS

The task of diagnosing a health problem is often a challenging bit of detective work, requiring perseverance and creativity to solve the riddles of human pathophysiology and symptomatology. While some patients and families received a medical diagnosis quite early in their chronic illness experience, the more common situation involved a lengthy and frustrating search for answers. For those who experienced it, a lengthy diagnostic testing process was powerful in shaping the way that the patient and family understood and experienced the illness thereafter. The accounts of these men and women about this process reveal typical encounters with health care that foreshadow those that will become prominent in the later discussions of chronic illness experience.

The long and complex process by which one young woman came to be diagnosed with MS reveals the frustration of trying to solve a diagnostic puzzle. Myrna's first signs at age 20 were "tingling and numbness in the feet," which kept "climbing higher and higher." She also experienced temporary loss of vision in one eye from time to time over several years. Her family doctor and optometrist did not seem overly concerned, but would offer reassurance and propose a variety of theories about what might be causing her symptoms. Finally, at the age of 26, she insisted on neurological tests. In this case, the patient instigated much of the detective work herself.

Even when the patient was under appropriate medical care, however, the process could be equally tortuous. Catherine's father became ill and was hospitalized with cardiac symptoms in a small town some distance from her home. On Catherine's behalf, a relative requested a transfer to the city hospital, but was told such measures were unnecessary. Her father was released 3 weeks later without a formal diagnosis or treatment. On discharge, he collapsed on the sidewalk two blocks from the hospital and was readmitted. Again, the family waited. Two weeks later, they discovered that the father's file had been lost in the computer, and the formal transfer request had never been sent. The cases of both Myrna and Catherine illustrate that, from the informants' perspective, the diagnostic process involves much more than just analyzing the results of tests. Rather, attracting sufficient attention within the health care system to have the tests performed in the first place can be an even more challenging aspect of the process.

Contrary to the expectations of many chronically ill patients and their families, the long process of diagnostic testing did not guarantee a definitive conclusion. For one young woman, a full year of invasive diagnostic procedures brought no answers.

> So [the doctor] had phoned, in fact, to say that he was sorry that he didn't know of anything else that he could do at the moment, and would I come back in a year. And I started to cry, because, through all those testing and that, I was feeling worse and worse. . . . And then for him to phone and say to come and see him in a year, well, it was just—I'm not a crybaby, but I'd had enough. I was upset.

Like many others, this woman had assumed that medical diagnosis is a complex but rigorous scientific process which continues until it has been successful. However, the degree to which guesswork figured in the process was a shock to many patients and families.

> People would say, "Well, maybe you have MS," or "Probably you have MS," or "In all likelihood you might have MS," or "It could be that," and they line up a whole ton of X-rays, and then they didn't like those X-rays, and they whipped me back for more!

Another woman remembered being offered an incredible range of rather unscientific explanations for her symptoms before her illness was finally diagnosed.

> One guy said, "Well, you probably have polio." The same one told me it could be arthritis. That was when I was 20. He said, "Well, you're not too young to have arthritis," and just named something. So far, no cancer that I know of! Oh, one guy said that I slept wrong, that's why I was going paralyzed! . . . I'm not making it up. I couldn't even make some of this stuff up!

Still others were quite stunned at the lack of scientific curiosity displayed by their professional health providers, as one woman's account illustrates.

> The doctor would take pictures, and would take blood tests, and when they don't find anything, then that's it! There's no curiosity, there's no, "Well, we're going to get to the bottom of this." There wasn't any inclination to dig.

Another complicating factor encountered by several of these people with chronic illness was what they regarded as misdiagnosis at some point in the process. One woman, who later turned out to have scleroderma, had been given a series of hot wax treatments for pain in her hands on the assumption that her problem might be arthritis. Her hands turned purple and became so swollen that "they felt like they were going to burst." For many patients and families, such misdiagnosis contributed to the extent of the eventual health problem. As the sister of one very ill young man wondered, "Maybe if the ulcer had been dealt with, it wouldn't have perforated . . . [and] he wouldn't have had pancreatitis, which is now a chronic problem."

While many of the chronically ill individuals and families blamed health care professionals for misdiagnoses, others accepted some measure of responsibility because of their eagerness to find a solution to their health care problem. On the advice of a specialist, Yvonne recalled agreeing to a tonsillectomy in the hopes that it would help her chronic sore throat and earaches. When the resident physician examined her the evening before the surgery, he noted that there was nothing apparently wrong with her tonsils. At her insistence, however, he reluctantly agreed to the operation, which later turned out to have a disastrous effect on the scleroderma that was eventually diagnosed. While this woman's account clearly demonstrates the desperation she felt at the time, it also suggests a lack of real leadership from her professional medical advisers.

For many patients and families, a telling feature of the diagnostic testing process was having their symptoms minimized or ignored by health professionals. Many recalled being told that their symptoms were purely psychological, as one woman with Inflammatory Bowel Disease (IBD) recalled.

> In 1965, I started complaining of stomach problems and I would just be told I was a nervous person and took things too seriously—just the usual line that people receive—women probably particularly, you know—that they overreact. And all this time there were numerous X-rays and then looking at the stomach with barium and so on. And I was just always told that I was a neurotic type (*laugh*) . . . and perhaps my job as a teacher was too much for me. And probably I was one of these people who was all too anxious to do well with everything, you know, and be an overachiever.

Another woman received a similar message from her professional health care providers.

> [Myasthenia Gravis] came on when my son was being born. . . . You know, anything affecting nerves and muscles for a myasthenic is bad. So I was in

a [myasthenic] crisis when I came out of the anesthetic. . . . They sent in a neurologist who did a few taps, you know, no blood work, no nothing. He was in my room, I think, 5 minutes, and he left, and said, "You know, she's a young mother—first baby. It's all in her head." Hysterical paralysis is what he called it.

The message that it was "all in their heads" was implied in other cases in which patients were actually admitted to psychiatric inpatient units for the purpose of diagnostic testing. One woman described being placed on "the psycho ward" for neurological testing. While she resisted being identified with the mentally ill, others found the opinion of others triggered doubts about their own sanity. One woman's account of the early stages of MS illustrates:

I sort of had a nervous breakdown, and terrible depression for a year, and I ended up seeing a psychiatrist, and when I was in there talking to him I'd say, "I'm sorry, I have to go to the bathroom." And often my husband was sitting there with me when we were talking, and he'd say to my husband, "Oh, just talking about it makes her want to go," you know. So I began thinking it was all up here, all this bladder business, 'cause every time I walked 10 feet I had to go to the bathroom. Yeah, well, it's typical medical profession. They couldn't really solve it. I began to think it was all in my head too, of course.

Thus, for many of the informants, the diagnostic testing process was an intensely difficult and confusing time, characterized by serious doubts about the benevolence or competence of health professionals as well as questions about their own sanity. However, in spite of such hurdles, the persistence of the informants was quite remarkable. As one explained, "You're always thinking, well, maybe they've got a magic pill somewhere." The hope that some solution to the health problem was right around the corner sustained many of these people through an astoundingly frustrating quest for a diagnosis.

THE DIAGNOSTIC EVENT

Being diagnosed featured prominently in the accounts of most of the chronically ill individuals and families in this study. Two distinct patterns in the diagnosis event were evident. For many, this event was experienced as a moment in time, that moment at which the chronic illness was given a name, and that moment at which the future was sealed. For others, there was no such moment, but rather a series of events during which the patient's identity and future were negotiated.

For some of the patients and families, the diagnosis emerged gradually in keeping with a predicted course of events. For example, one woman described the gradual process of realizing that her back problem would be permanent as "slow torture." In others cases, diagnosis was pronounced, withdrawn, and revised over time in accordance with changes in the patient's condition. As one woman with MS commented, "You see, it's hard to tell, because it's been sort of diagnosed, and then not diagnosed. People keep retracting, and then diagnosing." Another woman described a similar period of confusion around her diagnosis with arthritis.

> Rheumatologists are very strange people. They first of all tell you, like that, that I didn't have it. And then another time when I would be denying it, you know, doing a lot of things that they thought I shouldn't, they said that I was not being realistic and accepting it.

For such informants, each change in the diagnostic status brought new hopes and expectations, new questions and worries.

Some of the informants experienced a more gradual recognition process which they later attributed to their own inability to incorporate the information all at once. One woman, for example, recalled needing some time before the diagnosis could sink in.

> Part of it was not wanting to believe it. Like a bit of denial so that I didn't want to know too much more about it, because it really wasn't that bad, but once it started really getting bad, then I wanted to know more about it.

Thus, when inaccurate or incomplete information was available, or when the individual postponed accepting the importance of the impact of illness, the diagnostic event could be a slow and gradual process.

For most patients and families, however, one of the more profound and vivid memories in the chronic illness story was that moment at which they were given their diagnosis. For some, this diagnosis was expected. One young man recalled being finally told that his condition was incurable. "I was kind of shocked. Not shocked in a way, but shocked to hear it in reality, 'cause I knew there was something wrong, but just to hear it come out in reality was a shock for me." For others, the diagnosis came as a complete surprise. One woman's unexpected diagnosis with MS during pregnancy reflects such an experience.

> I said, "Well, surely there's a name for this," and he said, "Yes, it's Multiple Sclerosis." I was literally dumbfounded! I couldn't then speak. It was stunning! . . . For all intents and purposes, I was hearing it for the first time. I was hearing it directed at me. The only thing that I was able to say—like I say, I was dumbfounded literally. I said, "Is it serious?" and he said, "Yes, it's serious." . . . So I presumed that yes, I was . . . terminal.

For 6 hellish weeks, this woman's belief that she was dying, was imminently terminal, was not corrected. Whether it was anticipated or not, the moment of hearing the actual diagnosis was often experienced as profoundly shocking and disturbing. However, the urgency and anxiety with which people experienced the diagnosis event often went unrecognized by the health care professionals involved. Many patients and families explained that the timing and setting of the diagnosis were of major significance. One woman vividly recalled, for example, the overly casual context in which the devastating news of her son's cardiac condition was delivered.

> Saturday morning, I arrived at the hospital. And Dr. P. arrived in his jogging suit, with his little girl, and proceeded to stand in the hallway and tell me that they felt there was nothing that they could do for him because they couldn't get a shunt in. So, basically, it was fatal.

Richness of detail also betrayed the importance of certain terms or prognostications included in the information given to patients and families at the time of diagnosis. The account of one woman, on discovering that her newborn daughter suffered from PKU (Phenylketonuria), is one such example.

> He explained it very well, but the only thing I remember about that interview was the word "mental retardation," you know. As soon as that word came out, that was the word that stuck, and no matter how many times he said, "She's gonna be okay as long as she stays on the diet," and, you know, "these kids are fine," I didn't believe it. All I was thinking of, was a Mongoloid child, was what I could visualize in my mind.

In another mother's memory, the events surrounding the diagnostic event were equally vivid. After some months of exhibiting relatively mild digestive and respiratory symptoms, Maria's child was diagnosed with Cystic Fibrosis (CF).

> The only thing I know about Cystic Fibrosis—which was pretty well zip—was that we have a friend who lost a daughter to it many years ago . . . and when he told me this, I absolutely went to pieces! I was wringing my hands, literally wringing my hands, as I was talking to him. And I was shaking like a leaf. I can recreate it in my mind. I start to cry when I think about it.

Maria waited until her young children were asleep that night before sharing the news with her husband. As she recalled, "He damn near went crazy. . . . We cried all night." Not until the next day, when she barged in to her family doctor's office in a hysterical state, was Maria given any indication that treatment might allow her child to live.

In many such instances, the individuals involved felt as if the world had stopped at the moment of diagnosis and that life would never be the same. Their heightened sensitivity to the scene around them, to such details as the time of day and the sequence of conversation, suggests a great deal about how vivid and painful the diagnosis memories can be. Further, in each case, there was evidence that many of the professional health care providers had no inkling of the profound existential crisis their information had provoked. Thus, for many informants, the moment of telling took on great significance as a pivotal event in the chronic illness experience.

THE MEANING OF DIAGNOSIS

While the preceding illustrations suggest something of the intensity of the diagnosis event, they do not fully reveal the range of meaning it held for various patients and their families. In the following discussion, the meaning of diagnosis will be examined in relation to accounts of what the illness experience was like prior to diagnosis and, consequently, how the diagnosis altered that experience. In addition, the accounts will contrast such meanings with the informants' interpretations of what the diagnoses seemed to mean to the health care professionals involved.

For many informants, the most important meaning of the diagnostic event was that it brought a long and frustrating diagnostic process to an end. One woman's recollections epitomized the thoughts and feelings many associated with that process. She explained that, throughout the diagnostic process, she was unsettled by vacillating between hope that a minor and treatable disorder would be diagnosed and expectation that the diagnosis would be a terminal condition such as cancer. As she said, "That's always in your mind, when nobody's finding anything." In such cases, the process of worrying and hoping could end only if a diagnosis was made.

As has been noted, the diagnostic process often represented a threat to the patients' credibility in the eyes of others. According to several of these men and women, their integrity was in question as soon as diagnostic procedures failed to discover the problem. As one woman remembered, "So everything pointed to the fact, because technology couldn't point out why I had it at this point, that it had to be in my head." Another explained how this challenge to her credibility had discouraged her from pursuing a diagnosis for some time.

> I had been back to the doctor maybe three, four times, complaining of the aching, and I'd just get that skeptical look, like, you know, "Well, tension can do these things, and stress can do these things." . . . And I knew that there was something wrong, and I wasn't a hypochondriac . . . so I just stopped going to the doctor. And I didn't go to the doctor then for another couple of years.

When they could not get health care professionals to validate the health problem by giving it a diagnosis, the patients had a very difficult time explaining their illness to others in their family and social worlds. For example, one woman attributed the breakup of her marriage to the absence of such a confirming diagnosis.

> So through all this, my being tired and sore, and complaining, and worn out, and all that, and my marriage started to get into trouble, and finally my husband and I broke up. . . . I didn't even have anything to blame it on. It was like I was lazy, I didn't want to do anything, I couldn't participate, you know. . . . That was such a frustration, because I didn't know what was wrong.

As mentioned earlier, many patients and their families considered the diagnosis to be a critical turning point in their lives. For example, one young woman remembered being diagnosed with arthritis. "It was devastating. . . . It wasn't the plans so much it was me saying good-bye to a certain part of my life. 'Cause I knew . . . that I would have to change my life-style." For others, the event signaled the end of a different sort of crisis—the dilemma of having no explanation for their symptoms. For such individuals, the time of diagnosis could be experienced as a tremendous relief, as one woman's recollections of her diagnosis with Scleroderma illustrate.

> After being sick, or knowing there was something wrong, for nearly 17 years, I got a diagnosis of Progressive Systemic Sclerosis, which I had never heard of. But I was so excited, I was so thrilled for this man to be telling me I had this disease! It was stupid, you know—to have an answer. It didn't matter that it is a potentially fatal disease. None of that stuff mattered!

Another individual's account illustrates the encouraging effect that even a disturbing diagnosis could have on the illness experience in general. He remembered the diagnosis of his son's Cerebral Palsy (CP) this way:

> Even though the news was bad, I felt bloody relieved because at least I knew something, you know. We knew all those 6 months that there was something wrong. But we couldn't seem to get an answer. . . . And, you know, really, from that very next day we were home, [my wife] and I started to get along better, we started to talk about it, and talk to each other.

Another woman, also diagnosed with a serious and debilitating disease, explained how the diagnosis delivered her from an almost suicidal despair.

> And then I finally decided I'd do myself in, but I'd see one more psychiatrist. Thank God, I did! I was in his office, I think, 10 minutes, and he said there was nothing mentally wrong with me at all. He sent me, that afternoon, to a neurologist that he knew and within an hour they had me diagnosed as a Myasthenic. It was fantastic! I was so excited (*laugh*). I went to a party and celebrated (*laugh*). . . . So when the diagnosis came through I was ecstatic! I was thrilled! I had this rare neurological disease, and I was thrilled to pieces! Absolutely thrilled.

Without an appreciation for the profoundly traumatic effects of undiagnosed illness and of the diagnostic process itself, such enthusiastic reactions to devastating diagnoses would surely seem irrational.

The meaning of the diagnosis, therefore, was often contained in its reassuring implications that patients had not been manufacturing symptoms or exaggerating their case.

> When I said to Dr. G. not long ago, "Then this is a real problem, this is nothing I have just fooled around and invented, I mean this is a real problem?" And he said, "Hell, yes." Well that just like made me certified, you know (*laugh*). . . . She's got a legitimate problem. And I felt so good about having a problem that could be identified. I'd as soon not have the problem, quite honestly, but just to know that I haven't been malingering for the last 2 years!

Its meaning was also signified in its symbolic message of hope. As one man remarked, diagnosis gives you "a choice and a chance." Because there was a term for the problem and a reference point once diagnosis had been made, patients and families felt that "at least we're finally in action. It means doing something about the problem. It means that you're not just left alone." In addition, having a diagnosis helped people begin to come to terms with what had happened to them and to accept responsibility for what would follow. As one informant theorized:

> Somehow we can accept illness, especially if you know a definition for it. Originally it was very gratifying to know something was wrong with me. You get—if they were saying you were dying tomorrow, you'd be almost glad to hear it because it would give some sort of definite idea. It wouldn't be vague and lost and thinking you are responsible.

Thus, the meaning of the diagnosis for the patient and family seemed quite dependent on what their chronic illness experience had entailed prior to diagnosis. For those who had not experienced significant distress to that point, the diagnosis of a chronic condition could be profoundly disturbing, a major life crisis. However, among those whose prediagnosis experience had been lengthy, frustrating, and invalidating, the diagnosis often signified a welcome emancipation.

In contrast to their own experience, the patients and families in this study understood diagnosis to have a different set of meanings for the health care professionals involved in their care. Their thoughts on such meanings clearly reflect their interpretations of the behavior of such professionals over time throughout the diagnostic testing process.

Although the diagnosis represented the possibility of finally taking some action from the patient and family's point of view, many found that their health care professionals lost interest in their case once the diagnosis deemed the condition to be chronic. One man with MS observed:

> I may be all wrong in this, but my own opinion is, it's hard for the doctors to deal with, 'cause they can't do anything about it. . . . So they sort of do the tests, and sort of just turn the page, and get onto something else we can do something about, and sort of get rid of this, because we can't do anything about it.

Others also reported being disillusioned on discovering that the professionals' enthusiasm for the diagnostic process was not matched by an enthusiasm for helping patients cope with illness. As one woman recalled, the diagnosis seemed to signal a scientific dead end.

> It doesn't make a hill of beans of difference, because there's nothing you can do about it. Not a damned bit of good. It really doesn't. Maybe had they told me that many years ago, many, many years ago, you know, I might have understood. But there's so much damage—this kind of damage, psychological, and all these kind of damages that have been done along the way.

For many of these patients and families, the fact that the diagnosis produced little useful direction was a completely unanticipated occurrence. Some of them theorized, however, that this lack of direction might explain why their health care professionals had seemed so reluctant to diagnose chronic problems in the first place.

With the discovery that others experiencing similar disorders had undergone comparable difficulties in the prediagnostic phase, many patients and families were convinced that professionals had more difficulty with the idea of chronic illness than they did. Some theorized that the professionals were especially distressed by the idea that there was no cure. Others surmised that professionals avoided what they thought would be bad news. For example, having failed to obtain information from the physicians in charge, one woman recalled cornering a resident physician.

> And so I just said to him, I said, "Look," I said, "enough of this bullshit, let's get down to the bottom line here. What's going on?" So he just said, you know, "Look, if it's what we think it is, and to the extent that it is," he said, "[your son] is in serious trouble." So I said, "Thank you," you know, "for being honest with me."

Still others began to suspect that the whole diagnostic process might be marred by uncertainty, as one woman's story illustrates.

They don't know what to do, and they're just using B.S. I know that. Sure, I figured that out a long time ago. I've had it diagnosed many times, and then they go back and they say, "Well, maybe." . . . I went down [to the rehabilitation hospital] diagnosed, and came out being un-diagnosed. I went walking out there, and wheeled out in a wheelchair. Okay? It's completely opposite to what should happen.

Thus, many patients and families attributed the professionals' reluctance to diagnose chronic illnesses to an unconscious desire to avoid unpleasant realities and maintain hope that the health problem might spontaneously disappear.

A final clue to the meaning that diagnosis held for health professionals came from the patients' and families' observations that the existential significance of their diagnosis was often minimized or disregarded in the flurry of events. One woman's experience illustrated a particularly dehumanizing episode.

Right after I was diagnosed, a couple of days later, I received a paper like this in the mail. Would I please sign for the autopsy? Oh, yeah! I wish I'd kept it, you know. People don't believe it. I got very angry, I know, because I was having a little trouble with this whole problem. And I thought that was kind of tacky!

Such experiences led many patients and families to conclude that daily exposure to disease might have desensitized professionals to the importance of the diagnosis for the individual involved.

In general, then, the chronically ill individuals and their families came to understand that health care professionals were quite reluctant to diagnose a chronic health problem and, further, were often incapable of appreciating the significance of such a diagnosis to the patient and family. Thus, they came to recognize that a variety of meanings could be embedded in the diagnosis itself. Further, they began to appreciate that those meanings were often radically different for patients and their families than they were for health care professionals.

REPERCUSSIONS OF THE DIAGNOSIS

The accounts revealed that diagnosis was of particular importance in helping the patient and family accept and understand what had happened to them since the onset of disease. The most profound repercussion for many patients and families was an immediate and urgent need for information. As many explained, being left without sufficient information made the diagnosis of a chronic disease far more stressful than was necessary.

> You can't just dump something like that on someone, and these stupid little magazines, and just walk off. You can't do that! There's a million questions. You need support. You need someone you talk to. You need more!

Another patient agreed that information at such a time was essential.

> You get a bit stoned when you hear this kind of information. I really didn't know what Crohn's was, except that I was told now you've got it you've got it forever. . . . I had no conception of what it was. And I did not ever receive that information.

For many patients and families, information about the diagnosis and its meaning in personal terms was requisite to learning how to cope with a chronic illness. As one man explained:

> I can face up to things if somebody will tell me the truth. . . . I don't know if everyone's like that, but I've got to know, as much as I might get upset at the time. If you just tell me, then I'll deal with it, and go along from there.

Like this man, many found that their immediate need for information was pressing and unmet. As one father described it, "We were left entirely standing in the wilderness to find our own way."

While almost all of the chronically ill individuals and families in this study described a burning need for practical information upon diagnosis, several acknowledged that there were limitations to the information that was useful in the immediate aftermath. For example, a woman whose daughter had been diagnosed with PKU believed that professionals' admonishments about the possibility of mental retardation may have been cruelly excessive.

> I think they have to be honest, but I don't think they have to really push the retardation. Like with PKU, they push it so strongly, and it's so unfair. It is a fact that PKUs will be retarded without diet, but you have to realize that they're normal babies, too, and that's where it gets lost.

Similarly, many people complained that the information they had been given was inappropriate to their particular needs, thereby causing further undue distress. The recollections of one man illustrate:

> We went to the doctor, and then he said, "Well, of course you'll need insulin." Well, I just associated it with being a junkie of some sort! I couldn't get any sense out of that. . . . And then they gave me one manual, written in about 1912, and it said that most people with diabetes lose their legs and their vision, and their kidneys go, and that was it!

Recognizing that information-giving was a judgment call, one woman explained that health care professionals held stereotypes as to what information patients probably needed.

> I can understand now their prejudices, because they're in a whole different world than I was, and they had the knowledge, and if they start talking to me in their language, they figured I wouldn't know what they were talking about anyway, so why even bother explaining to me.

Because it was not forthcoming from the professionals, a number of the patients and families in this study took immediate action to acquire the necessary information. In fact, their resourcefulness and creativity in this regard was astounding, as one man's experience illustrates.

> After the surgery, I went around and I read everything I could get my hands on about Inflammatory Bowel Disease. . . . I'd get into libraries up at [the university], and went to [a major hospital library] and got in there. Nobody asked me any questions. I just went in, and started reading books. . . . And after I read it all, and I got all this knowledge, and stuff, I kind of put it out of my head, and got on with living again. . . . I had to know what I was up against before I felt okay about it. And I knew I wasn't gonna get it from the doctors.

Other chronically ill individuals and families were less skilled at meeting their information needs without help, as one woman's recollection illustrates.

> I felt alone in the world. There was no support whatever from the neurologist, from the family doctor. I didn't know anybody who knew anything about MS . . . and it was something I wasn't comfortable asking about it. It felt like a shoe that wasn't broken in yet . . . didn't fit.

Thus, people newly diagnosed with a chronic illness explained that the need for information was closely associated with finding ways to accept or cope with the their disease.

Beyond stimulating an urgent need for information, the immediate repercussions of the chronic illness diagnosis included dramatic adaptations for some patients and families. In some families, the diagnosis triggered profound feelings of loss and grieving. As one woman recalled: "I cried buckets. You go through this stage of feeling sorry for yourself, 'Why did it happen to me? What's the use of anything?' " In some families, the emotional distress triggered serious disruptions. As one woman recalled, "My husband asked for a divorce. He couldn't handle the illness. I don't blame him. If I could've walked out on me, I would've." One young man felt a particularly acute need to express his emotions through art.

> I started to draw, because I was getting so afraid of everything around me.
> I started to draw like crazy. And the drawings I did were so expressionistic.
> I was drawing animals fighting, and big, huge storms, and buildings
> exploding. . . . I look at them now, and it must've been a shock to some
> people, 'cause I would draw dead bodies, and I would draw people just
> lying all over the place, just dying, and stuff like that. Morbidity was really
> high, and I didn't think I was gonna live very long. And that was a part of
> the way of how I was accepting it.

His story reflects the extent to which managing the emotional turmoil was an essential element in coming to a sense of acceptance.

For the informants in this study, therefore, diagnosis of a chronic illness had immediate and serious repercussions for emotional and family life, and stimulated an urgent need for understanding what had occurred.

DISCUSSION

From the accounts of the patients and families in this study, it is evident that the onset and diagnosis of a chronic illness are profoundly influential in a person's life. Analysis of the help-seeking process as articulated in the scholarly literature confirms the informants' contention that the relationship between onset of illness and diagnosis is of critical importance to those involved (Chrisman & Kleinman, 1983;

McKinlay, 1981b). In addition, the research on chronic illness experience substantiates that the events associated with onset and diagnosis are often prolonged and traumatic for the patient and for the family (Corbin & Strauss, 1988). With few exceptions, the scholarly literature tends to consider these phenomena as if they are almost inevitable outcomes of the disease. Rarely does it consider the extent to which these experiences are twisted and molded by the peculiarities of health care encounters along the way. From the accounts of these informants, however, the role that health care plays in creating a straightforward or a tortured diagnostic process seems quite evident.

According to Mishler (1981), the medical diagnosis is far from an exact and scientific process. Common understanding assumes that diseases are "real entities," and that problems ascertaining the presence or absence of a disease in any given case are reflections of the state of progress in medical science. However, in actual practice, such precision is rarely the case, as is evident from numerous studies questioning diagnostic reliability. Rather, medical diagnoses can be better understood as constructions of a social reality within the context of a given set of assumptions, norms, and institutional requirements (Morgan et al., 1985). In Western cultures, they give biomedical meanings to human predicaments regardless of the degree to which the predicament is biomedically understandable (Duval, 1984).

A perspective such as this informs our understanding of why the diagnostic process may be as complex and as distressing as these informants claim it to be. Although a great many of the diseases represented in this study are poorly understood in biomedical terms, the processes and procedures by which professionals conduct the diagnostic testing are grounded in the assumption that identification of specific causes will produce specific remedies (Armstrong, 1983). Unfortunately, while the professionals are proceeding according to the book, the patients' conditions fail to cooperate, making the potential for misunderstanding and insensitivity extreme. Thus, the onset and diagnosis of chronic illness are experiences that may be best appreciated within the context of the social conditions that shape them, primarily those within the health care arena.

Acuity and Chronicity

Chronic illness takes various forms, exerting a range of influences upon the life of the individual and the family afflicted. Chronicity, or the state of being chronically ill, constitutes a collection of states that share common elements. According to the accounts of the patients and families in this study, some of these include a realization process, extensive maintenance work, accounting for acute episodes, and an eventual acceptance of chronicity. From their perspective, these elements make chronic illness, in all of its various patterns, quite distinct from the acute episodic illness that is expected throughout the life cycle.

PATTERNS OF CHRONICITY

The patients and families in this study revealed that there were a variety of distinct patterns in which chronic illness unfolded. One such pattern was the gradual progression of symptoms over an extended period of time, as one woman's experience with arthritis illustrates:

> I've had it over 20 years but, like, the first 10 or 12, they were quite tolerable. I wasn't crippled. I got around quite well and all that. And then, bit by bit, I lost a finger (*laugh*) and now both my hips are replaced. In fact one of them's been done twice.

While surgical intervention would have rendered her incapacitated for brief periods of time over those 20 years, the effects of the disease were almost imperceptible over time, their course characterized by few sudden changes and a fairly predictable progression. Another patient remembered the gradual process of her illness.

It's been very slow. When I was diagnosed it was just a bad limp. There was nothing wrong, nothing. They couldn't see a thing. Then it was '72, and that was the point where I started to go downhill. It was like I had a so-called attack—they're spaced further apart now, but at one point I was nearly blind, and a lot of times I hadn't been able to walk very well.

For this woman, the slow progression was demarcated not by surgical interventions, but by acute episodes in her illness.

Other informants experienced a pattern characterized by a series of changes followed by a gradual stabilization of symptoms. One woman described the pattern of her chronic neck pain as cycles of suffering for 3 or 4 weeks followed by a period in which the discomfort was more like a "subtle presence." In contrast, some people experienced diseases characterized by dramatic changes in course. One man's description suggests the frustration inherent in such an illness pattern.

There's so many ups and downs with this Crohn's. . . . You start to build up, you're having a good time, you think you've got your life in order a little bit and whammo! You're back in again, major surgery, and you start recovering again. . . . Yeah, it takes a fair amount out of you emotionally. There's no doubt about it.

While these conditions are all chronic in nature, such different patterns reveal dramatically different effects on the degree to which life can be planned, the speed with which changes must be confronted, and the extent to which new frustrations are layered upon the old.

While each disease entity tended to have its own pattern of chronicity, patients and families discovered that the pattern was also unique to each individual involved. As one patient explained, IBD is "such a disease of variables. I mean, from the mildest form and a one-attack, to people that have a chronic, and sometimes acute. And it's so different with every patient." In some cases, the disease offered the dangling carrot of remission, a period during which symptoms subside. Yet, because remission itself could be quite unpredictable, it too became a frustrating feature of chronic illness, as one informant's recollections illustrate.

I said, "You know, when is it ever gonna get better?" I mean, I had done a lot of reading at this point, and I knew that, you know, the disease should go into remission, or that's what everybody had hoped. And [my doctor] said, "Well, it might not get a whole lot better." Well, I really started panicking at this, because I wasn't even coping—taking care of the family.

For this woman, as for others, the realization that there was no such thing as "going by the book" was an important aspect of understanding the pattern of chronicity. In general, learning to manage required discovering one's unique pattern rather than depending upon generalized predictions about the disease.

For some patients, the unpredictable ups and downs of chronic illness were its most frustrating feature. One informant described her MS as unpredictable in this way:

> It's horrible! It comes and goes, it comes and goes, it teases me every once in a while. Sometimes I'm just like a normal person, and another time I'm just—well, they hauled me out of here in an ambulance 2 weeks ago. Totaled. Completely finished. Totaled. Couldn't walk, couldn't do anything. I was gone.

For others, the unrelenting permanence of symptoms made chronic illness most difficult to tolerate. As one young man remarked, "Any human being could cope with it for half an hour." Having to cope with it permanently, however, was an entirely different proposition.

Whatever the pattern of chronicity or degree of predictability, however, these chronically ill patients and families all confronted changes as a result of having a chronic disease. Their life-styles and future plans became dependent upon conditions of the body that were, to some degree, beyond their control. What made them different from well people was that they recognized the degree to which bodily health is always fragile and unpredictable. Even periods of relative health could present problems, as one woman's thoughts illustrate.

> You are not prepared for health. . . . Suddenly a door opens, and you have a world in front of you that you never had before. You really don't know how to deal with it. And then, there's the nagging thing that is always in the background. You know it may not last. And of course, we all know that things are not necessarily permanent, but with a chronic condition, you have less concept of permanency.

The concept of "illness trajectory" has been proposed in the literature as a means by which to conceptualize such variations in the pattern of chronic illness. According to the proponents of this concept, symptoms alone do not explain the experiential progressions that characterize the pattern of chronic illness. Rather, such features as the work involved in being chronically ill, the organization of such work, and the impact of the work on the people involved are all considered significant to the way that chronic illness enacts itself in individual lives (Corbin & Strauss, 1988; Strauss & Corbin, 1988; Strauss et al., 1984). Symptom severity and fluctuation create conditions in which the work of illness may or may not be manageable, and produce circumstances in which the patient and family may or may not be able to mobilize resources to plan effectively.

In considering the notions of acuity and chronicity in the context of the chronic illness experience, there are a range of possible trajectories. The accounts of these informants provide an important window into our understanding of what chronicity and acuity have to do with shaping both this trajectory and the overall meaning this experience has for them. Further, they provide another illustration of the degree to which the chronic illness experience is inherently influenced by the way in which disease necessitates health care involvement in our society.

COMING TO TERMS WITH CHRONICITY

The onset and/or diagnosis of a chronic condition set in motion a process by which the patients and families came to terms with what chronic illness entailed and what it meant to be chronically ill. This process involved not only learning the particular pattern of disease progression that the illness would take, but also included making sense of the social context in which the chronic illness would be lived.

Realization that the illness would be an ongoing component of their lives was a slow and gradual process for most of these informants. As one explained, "At first when it was diagnosed, there was sort of a period of denial." Another described gradual recognition of the meaning of having a chronic illness.

> For a long time I was making very unrealistic goals. I mean, I came back saying, "Oh, yeah, I got a little bronchitis here, my asthma's a little nutsy, I'll take a few antibiotics and I'll be through this." And as that winter progressed, I mean, I was just constantly making inappropriate goals for myself, you know. . . . So I went through a big frustration just in the sense that I was nowhere near coming to accept that this was a chronic illness.

For many, the information obtained at the time of diagnosis was insufficient to help them absorb the very real implications of the illness.

Recognition of chronicity, therefore, tended to be a gradual process, in which various implications of the illness were realized at different times and with different degrees of difficulty.

Interpreting People's Responses

The individuals and families in this study found that chronic illness provoked a peculiar set of responses from people in their social worlds. For many, figuring out the meaning of these responses was central to understanding the implications of chronic illness. For those whose illness began with an acute episode, there was a point of comparison with which to gauge how people respond to illness that is chronic. One teacher, for example, remembered how helpful and cooperative people were in the initial phases, before his injury had become chronic.

> People were really understanding about that. . . . They let me use the school van because it's an automatic, and my car was a standard. . . . They all gave me lots of time, and lots of space. . . . It was just understood that I would be a little bit late for class, and I'm going to lie down on the couch, and I'm going to deliver my lecture lying down, because I can't get around that much. And that was okay. That was really well accepted.

However, that early tolerance was time-limited, and eventually these special privileges were no longer extended. As he learned, the social meaning of chronic illness was clearly much different from that of acute, short-term health problems.

Losing the ability to generate their own livelihood was the point at which the full impact of social attitudes toward the chronically ill hit home for many informants. Among the most humiliating and demeaning social experiences described was the attempt to obtain a handicapped pension or long-term disability allowance. According to one man, such a pension was the only possible means to an acceptable life with a serious chronic illness. As he recalled, "I was really suicidal. I thought I would just die if I can't get it, because I'm not gonna live like this." In many cases, chronically ill individuals believed that they were denied benefits to which they were legally entitled because of a general attitude of distrust toward the chronically ill. One man's account illustrates how frustrating it was to be suspected of malingering in order to obtain benefits.

> It makes you feel like nobody wants you. So you're a worker, big deal, forget it. We're not going to cover you, forget it. . . . You're wasting our

time. So, consequently, what is happening to me now is that I get up, and I'm going, "Oh yeah, I'm a degenerate. You know, I can't do this." Where before I'd just grab anything by the throat, go after it, and do it. But now I know always in the back of my mind, you know, my knees, my knees, my knees, you know. I'm always thinking about that. I can't do this, I can't do that. . . . So it's very frustrating . . . I can't go out and be a carpenter anymore.

Because they valued activity and employment so highly, the suggestion that they were exaggerating their symptoms in order to benefit from their illness was extraordinarily disturbing for many informants.

While unsympathetic attitudes from bureaucrats were frustrating, they were even more damaging when they surfaced among friends and families. To be fair, the vast majority of informants reported that families and friends were generous in their support and accepting in their attitudes. As one woman remarked, "My friends overwhelm me with kindness and love and attention, beyond anything that I deserve." However, some people discovered that having a chronic illness brought peculiar ideas and opinions out of the woodwork. One woman's experience coping with a sister's theory about her arthritis illustrates the distress that could result from such opinions.

And then my sister, who's a radical Christian, told me that she had asked God . . . why our mom had died. And God had told her it was because Mom didn't know enough of The Word, and therefore would I take these series of tapes she was going to give me, and would I learn The Word, so that I wouldn't also die like Mom did, because I didn't know enough of The Word, or something. And oh, that upset me so badly. I was thinking that she was really saying, "The reason for what you're having is that you aren't being enough of a believer."

While such attitudes among close friends and family could be devastating, the possibility that health care professionals might be less sympathetic to the chronically ill than to the acutely ill was an even more disturbing revelation, as one woman's experience illustrates.

If you have a chronic disease you're going about the same things all the time, and you can't help it because those same things flare time after time and when you go in. And the doctor looks at you like [*facial expression*]. It's not your imagination, it's a definite, "Oh, my God, here she is again" kind of thing, you know. You can tell by the expression.

Often, the difference in attitude appeared as soon as the illness was diagnosed as chronic. As one mother of a child with Cerebral Palsy (CP) observed, "Since [my son] wasn't a real critical patient any more, [the doctor] he had other things on his mind instead."

Informants offered various theories about such attitudinal shifts on the part of health care professionals. In the opinion of one woman, this attitude reflected a preference for patients who presented with "a hands-on thing that the doctor can deal with" such as "appendicitis" or a "deviated septum." In contrast, in chronic illness,

> All his little things don't work, his X-ray pictures don't work, and his blood tests and his urine tests don't work, and then that is a real problem to the doctor. . . . So, I guess the doctors want to see healthy people.

Another theorized that chronicity, because it represented neither health nor incapacitating illness, was particularly frustrating to her physicians.

> I'm sure they'll all be much happier if I . . . just blew my brains out, and died, you know, there'd be no problem, eh? Or if it exaggerated to the point where they had absolute control over me, okay, fine. But now that I'm in-between, they don't like it.

Others suspected that their health care professionals' disinterest reflected a more general disinterest in chronic conditions within medical science. One patient's angry comments illustrate such a suspicion. She said, "Come on, it's time! They're going to cure AIDS, or herpes, before they get to MS. The whole world is panicked over AIDS, right? Totally panicked. That's because some doctor must've got it."

Thus, one important dimension of the process of coming to terms with chronicity involved recognizing that unsympathetic social attitudes, including those of health professionals, would be an important part of the chronic illness experience.

Changing Expectations

Another element in the process of coming to terms with chronicity was changing expectations about their lives, their health, and their health care. Once diagnosis had been made and some idea of prognosis provided, patients and their families gradually recognized that a complete cure was unlikely. For many, this recognition was pivotal in their process of "getting on with life." As one woman commented, "I think now I don't expect the doctor to fix me up. I expected it when I was diagnosed."

For some patients and families, this shift from a cure to a care orientation was assisted by honesty from health care professionals with regard to what life with chronic illness would entail. However, such clear communication was not considered standard practice. In fact, many reported being devastated by negative or tactless remarks from health care professionals at that time.

> To me, what they should say is, "There's nothing we can do at this time, but there is research going on all the time, and hopefully in some years to come, there will be something for this disease," you know, instead of just flat saying, "There's nothing that can be done," period.

According to these patients and families, when health care professionals were faced with a situation for which there was no known cure, they appeared to give up. From the perspective of those living with chronic illness, this was an attitude too harsh to accept and too cruel to understand. For them, giving up was not an option. Once they accepted that a cure might not be possible, they aimed their sights at alternative goals, such as improved quality of life, symptom control, and productivity. Further, they often remained surreptitiously optimistic that a cure might someday be found. As one woman said, "I hope I'm in the right lineup when the Higher Power says, 'Okay, we're going to take asthma away from this number of people today.'" Another echoed, "Like, I'm not expecting a miracle, although if something happened I wouldn't mind."

Thus, coming to terms with chronicity required these patients and families to confront attitudes about chronic illness and about the potential for its cure. Such confrontations were conducted in the context of a social environment in which the opinions and beliefs of family, friends, authority figures, and health professionals were instrumental in shaping the everyday experience with chronic illness.

THE WORK OF CHRONICITY

Having a chronic illness required that the informants devote a considerable amount of energy toward maintaining their health status and managing their emotional stability, both of which have been referred to as the work of chronic illness (Corbin & Strauss, 1988). According to their accounts, coming to terms with chronicity required that they learn how to handle this work effectively. The following description will provide a subjective impression of how extensive this work can be and how great a burden it can represent.

Health Maintenance Work

These chronically ill individuals and families described much of their work in terms of maintaining the best level of health that they were able to achieve with chronic illness. Invariably, they struggled to maintain or to improve existing levels of strength, comfort, symptom control, weight, or mobility—whatever symbolized health in the context of their own disease. For many patients, energy conservation was among the most important components of health maintenance. Since fatigue is a well known effect of many chronic conditions, this priority was not surprising.

As has previously been pointed out, the lives of the chronically ill were not eclipsed by the illness; rather, illness tended to create an additional stressor within already complicated lives. Thus, patients and families described health maintenance as a juggling act in which each element contributed to the total performance. One woman's words depict the complexity of this juggling act for her.

> Learning can only begin to happen when you are well enough, or calm enough, or have enough nutrient in you for you to stop worrying about basic physical existence: What'll I eat today? Have I got enough money for the mortgage? Are the kids fed and clothed? Will I not have pain today? Simple little things. And only when you can begin to put some of those into some kind of context, where they're not the preoccupying thoughts of the day, can you begin to start to talk about learning what to do with them.

Although many people identified pacing and planning ahead as essential in managing the work of chronic illness, few found these skills easy to master. As one patient explained, "You don't know where your limits are, so you keep testing them all the time. It is like the child learning to walk, sometimes."

Prevention of acute episodes or health deterioration was another element of health maintenance work for these patients and families. In this regard, many reported being advised to remove stress from their lives. As one woman's criticisms suggest, this advice was often perceived as superficial and insulting.

There's no point in saying to someone like myself, "You mustn't live a stressed life," you know. I mean it's very hard to think of a metaphor, or a simile that you can use in saying you must now cease and desist from a stressed life. If I stop my university career, and go into hibernation some-where, the stresses of having given up something for nothing, with nothing to fill it, are going to be probably as stressful!

For many of those living with chronic illness, much of the work of preventing acute episodes included adhering to certain dietary, medi-cation, or exercise regimens prescribed by a health care professional. Again, this work required constantly juggling priorities to discover which of the requirements were personally applicable and which were not. Even when there was complete commitment to following the prescribed regimen to the letter, the actual work involved in doing so was often overwhelming. One mother's account illustrates a situation that was particularly taxing in the initial stages.

So we start off with this kid that's never swallowed a pill, and has to take five a day—that's the starters. She had to take one antibiotic, two pills, four times a day, and the other one, two pills three times a day, and the antibiotics weren't supposed to be taken close to the meals, you know—the usual. I mean, it's impossible. It can't be done, there's no way. Came home, I sat down with a piece of paper, and I had to write down every hour of the day, and I'd put in the [medications], and the vitamin, that was easy, and then I took those other ones, and tried to figure it out. It was like I was driving a jet plane, the dials, and all this, you know. It was so boggling, really.

In many cases, orchestrating coordinated services, preparing restricted diets, or managing regular therapy sessions presented these patients and families with an almost impossibly complex managerial assignment.

Thus the work of preserving the health they had; of protecting them-selves against the event of acute episodes, deterioration, or secondary effects; and of following treatment plans was significant for most of the patients and families in this study. For them, chronic illness was indeed very hard work!

Emotional Work

A second category of work articulated by these informants involved the work required to regulate their emotions, to protect themselves and their families against excessive depression or anxiety, and to prepare themselves for the fearful events that were anticipated in the course of the illness. This emotional work was described with at least as much passion and detail as was the health maintenance work, suggesting its significance in the overall scheme of things for these informants.

As would be expected, chronic illness confronted many people with a source of extreme emotional distress, particularly in the early stages. The recollections of one mother of a child with CF illustrate.

> At the beginning, I guess you're just absolutely wringing your hands and in tears all the time. You just can't bear that this is my daughter or even that it's happened. And after a while you start living with it. . . . You can't live in that intense state of worry, even for a year. I mean you couldn't go through your day if you're as worried as you were initially.

For many patients and families, the emotional roller coaster of chronic illness was driven by events in the illness, as one mother's experience suggests.

> I do just marvelously, because she's doing well. And as soon as she doesn't do well, everything falls apart. Like I just crumble right up. It's just like I'm back just starting all over again, trying to deal with it.

Others pointed to the unrelenting nature of their pain or discomfort as the central emotional trigger.

> I'm actually quite amazed how it's affected me . . . having that constant ache there, just can really make you teary-eyed. And sometimes I just think, "Oh, why doesn't this stress go away," you know? "Why doesn't it just go away?"

Life events secondary to the chronic illness could themselves become a major source of emotional distress, as one informant noted.

> A lot of people are coping with [illness using] liquor, and pot, and shrinks. They're coping day by day, just getting through. Oh, it's a horrible thing that's happening to people. Awful. They've lost husbands, they've lost wives, they've lost everything. . . . And they're perfectly nice, innocent people that just have circumstances.

Among the many emotional responses described by patients and families, self-pity was seen as particularly dangerous. As one individual remarked, "I know I could wallow in it if I wanted to. But you can't afford that luxury, I think, because you make yourself ill in the process." Another frighteningly common response to chronic illness was depression. As one man's account revealed, depression often resulted from disappointments about symptom management procedures.

> You see, there's always so many disappointments that there's a tendency to give up, because this thing that I'm trying to do—a new approach, a new doctor, a new something, and it doesn't work—then you just get depressed again. And because you counted on it, you had hoped that it was going to be improved. And when it didn't, then you just get depressed and down again.

Depression was also a common response to the losses associated with chronic illness, as another patient's comments illustrate.

> You know, I wanted to get married, I got married. I was so happy, I was ready for a family, and stuff like that. And it all went down the drain. And now you think, is it all worth it? Is everything worth it? And why did it happen to me?

In fact, many of the informants in this study reported episodes of depression so severe that they contemplated suicide or welcomed the possibility of death.

Another dimension of the emotional work described by many of these patients and families was dealing with fear and anxiety. Predictable changes in the course of the disease provided a focus for intense worry, as in the case of those who would someday become incapacitated by their disease. In other instances, preoccupation with possibilities for the future produced acute anxiety. The most vivid accounts of such anxieties came from parents concerned for the futures of their children. For example, one mother contemplated the worst case scenario for her daughter.

> You're so protective of your child. To lose her, I just—and it isn't even the losing of her. I don't even want her to suffer. Like I just couldn't bear for her to be in such desperate straits. The thought of her gasping, and choking for air—it paralyzes me. Like I cannot deal with that! I don't know how, if I ever have to deal with it—God, I hope I don't! I don't know how people deal with it.

While some patients and families found it helpful to avoid thinking about dreaded possibilities, others believed that being prepared for even the worst outcomes was essential to maintaining emotional health. For example, one woman turned to published autobiographical accounts as a source of information about what the worst outcomes might entail. Although she found them painful to read, she felt that she had to know the worst. "I don't think you should be kept totally in the dark, because then it's too much of a shock if things went wrong." The emotional work involved in chronicity, therefore, included a wide range of experiences in managing emotional distress, preventing depression, and overcoming anxieties about the future.

The accounts of these patients and families also featured the role that health care professionals played in either facilitating or inhibiting emotional work. Some people found individual health care providers to be excellent sources of support and guidance in this regard. However, a great many others reported that the attitudes and theories of the professional health care providers exacerbated the difficulties and made the emotional work more perplexing. For example, Margaret's attempts to provide emotional support to her depressed adult son with IBD put her in conflict with hospital staff.

> When I could see it was really bad, I thought well, I'll have to do something about this. I really braced myself when I'd go in. And I'd bawl him out. I would . . . tell him he came from a line of people that weren't people that gave up . . . I'd tell my son it wasn't in his genes to be a giver-upper, you know? And I wasn't gonna allow it . . . and we'd have a cry, and it would be all over.

Until Margaret realized that other IBD family members had successfully used similar strategies, she felt the sting of criticism from the hospital nurses and social worker acutely.

In addition to holding incompatible ideas about what ought to constitute the emotional work of chronic illness, many patients and families found health care professionals quite unsupportive of what chronically ill people were undergoing. One woman's description of interactions with her physiotherapist illustrates. As she observed, "She doesn't understand chronic illness. She upset me something awful. . . . I felt like a scolded child the whole time I was there." Such instances were unfortunately common in the experience of the informants and resulted in their frequent conclusion that health professionals did not particularly care. As one young woman said, "I don't think they really appreciate what it feels like to be chronic."

Thus, the accounts illustrate that chronicity is characterized by health maintenance and emotional work, and that this work is of major concern to chronically ill individuals and their families. They further point out the extent to which this work is carried on outside of formal health care, and, at times, is made more difficult by attitudes and beliefs originating within the health care system.

ACUTE EPISODES IN CHRONICITY

In some chronic illnesses, episodes in which the patient's health is more compromised than usual may occur. In other chronic illnesses, there are periods of time, such as surgeries, in which the patient's health status is radically altered. In yet other chronic illnesses, resistance is so low that the patient can suddenly become quite ill with such common "everyday" conditions as seasonal colds. As was evident from the discussion on patterns of chronicity, acute episodes are quite disruptive and disturbing for those involved. In this discussion, the accounts of informants will explain the meaning of acute episodes in the context of chronic illness, focusing on hospitalization as an especially problematic event.

Managing Acute Episodes

From the perspective of patients and their families, acute episodes were a dramatic departure from daily living with chronic illness. In an acute episode, symptoms were exaggerated or different, bodily cues were altered, and emotional reactions were extreme. The recollections of one young man with IBD are a dramatic illustration.

> One night, I remember I was in bed . . . and my heart started to pound . . . I thought I was gonna die. I really did, because my chest was pumping, my heart was going, and I looked down, and I couldn't believe it, that my chest could move out that far. And I figured it was gonna stop, instantly, in the next beat. The room started changing color, it went from orange, to red, and then to bright white, and I lay there going, "This is it. I'm gonna die."

For many people living with chronic illness, acute episodes also provided visible markers of disease progression. One woman, for example, found herself measuring her child's progress in terms of the length of time between hospitalizations. When he was hospitalized after 6 months instead of the predicted 18, "I thought holy—does this mean that's he's two-thirds as bad? Like sort of a mathematical formula you dig up for that."

Acute episodes required that patients and families relinquish the usual control they exerted over their lives and their health care. As one man explained, "The crisis takes over. And if it really is acute you are in no position to argue and negotiate." Informants explained the shift in control as something that they allowed to happen because of the emergency nature of the event. In addition, they agreed that assertiveness was extremely difficult when one was feeling sick. "I find that when you're really sick you're not in an argumentative mood. You don't feel strong within yourself. You just do, sort of, whatever anybody tells you to do."

Because they recognized their inability to remain in charge of decisions during an acute episode, many patients made arrangements for others to assist them in the event. One young man explained why he asked his parents to take charge during his acute episodes: "I can't look after myself, but I feel that I need somebody looking at me. I can't trust this hospital. . . . When I'm sick, I let people walk all over me." Given the distress that an acute health problem would naturally create for anyone, acute episodes in chronic illness were indeed frightening and anxiety producing. Further, because they induced a dependency that was quite different from patients' usual chronic illness work, such episodes were a highly disconcerting component of the chronic illness experience.

Dealing With Hospitalizations

For many patients and families, one of the most frightening features of an acute episode was that it placed them in a position of having to submit to hospitalization. As one man explained, "I didn't want to get exhumed (*sic*) into that system again." In many instances, fear of the hospital was the result of awareness that they could exert little control over who would look after them and the decisions they might make, as one woman's comments illustrate:

> I'm just hoping and praying to God that nothing happens that I will have to go to hospital, because I might get sent to [the local] hospital, and some knife-happy surgeon is gonna have me in the OR [operating room] before I can even blink an eye.

In addition, hospitals represented places where patients were often prohibited from carrying on their normal therapeutic regimens.

> I don't go into hospital and have them take my pills away. Never! Never! You know, doctors like to put you . . . on four-hour schedules, six-hour schedules, you know. Well, with Myasthenia you can't do that. I need my pills every hour—every hour, every 2 hours, sometimes every 7, you know. Who knows? I can't tell when. I just know inside me when I need to take them.

While losing control over the pacing and planning of daily routines was difficult for all patients, it seemed especially problematic for the parents of chronically ill children. One mother explained that, while in hospital, her 8-year-old was allowed to watch television programs she would have forbidden, stay up past his bedtime, and run wild in the corridors. "The kids are allowed a lot more freedom than they would have, you know, at home. . . . But it's not my house, you know. It's the hospital staff's house."

Adding to these problems of losing control, hospital experiences were often reminiscent of the time prior to diagnosis when patients had little idea of what was happening. In the hospital, they were often subjected to the whims of whatever health professionals happened to be on duty and to the routines by which the hospital functioned. Further, some patients and families believed that hospitals subjected them to additional health threats, such as secondary infections and complications from procedures. "You know how some people get in the hospital and they start with one thing and they wind up with a whole bunch of others."

According to many of these people, general hospitals were not planned with chronically ill people in mind. For example, one woman complained of how difficult it was for her to manage the beds in the general hospital.

> Now, if you go into a general hospital, they put the bed down, but it's still not low enough to stand there, and put your behind on the mattress. You have to step up onto a step stool to get into bed. . . . And especially for someone with MS, that's really wearing.

Others noted that while hospital staff were always eager to gather patient information, they were often less enthusiastic about applying it.

"I think why bother having this form, you know, if you're not going to attend to it."

Several of the patients and families believed that hospital staff tended to be particularly suspicious of chronically ill patients. In some cases, they claimed that nurses were "intimidated" by patients who "had been around awhile." For those who experienced repeated hospitalization, "learning the ropes" was critical.

> You know, even parking, in the hospital, I didn't know that you could pay your $3 and get a return thing, while I was paying every time I went in and out! You know, I was doing that for a week and a half before I found out, you know. And then we [parents] got the hang of it, so we were switching tickets off so that whoever was going out could come in with the next one.

Even when they had learned the ropes with regard to hospitalization, many patients and families found it difficult to protect themselves from its devastating effects. Because of this, many postponed hospitalization for as long as possible. When it became inevitable, others devised creative coping strategies. For example, Robert, a young man with IBD, claimed to dissociate for the duration of the hospitalization. "I just turn into nothing, you know. For a certain period of time, when I go into the hospital, I prepare myself in that this doesn't exist. It's not me. It's just a body they're gonna deal with."

The vivid descriptions that chronically ill individuals and their families gave of their experience with acute episodes reveals the extent to which such episodes influence life with a chronic illness. Acute episodes are often intensely dramatic and alter the control people exert over their lives and their health. It is difficult, therefore, to appreciate chronicity without an understanding of acuity in that context. For the chronically ill, it seems that acuity represents different challenges and conditions than it does for those in whom acute illness is a temporary aberration from a usual state of wellness.

ACCEPTANCE OF CHRONICITY

The accounts of the patients and families in this study suggest that the chronicity experience includes not only coming to terms with the fact of the illness but also, eventually, accepting that the illness has played and will continue to play a major role in shaping the lives of all concerned. According to many of these men and women, some form of acceptance was essential to getting on with life as a chronically ill person. One patient described it as "the ultimate decision to not worry about it anymore and just accept the fact that I'm a chronic."

For many of these patients and families, acceptance required considerable effort. However, their accounts often revealed a process whereby, after a time of struggle, acceptance came quite suddenly. One mother's recollection of accepting her child's chronic illness illustrates:

> Finally one day I just decided . . . I finally accepted him fully inside, to accept the way he is. But before that I really didn't. There was too much resentment, and stuff like that, in there.

Others found it to be a more gradual and evolutionary process. One man likened it to creating a new identity. "It took me 30 years to create a person, right? Now people expect you to get out of it in 2 years, so you have to find a new you."

For many patients and families, acceptance was greatly facilitated by honest information from health care professionals. In other cases, patients and families seemed to accept the illness before the health care professionals did. One young man's story illustrates such a case.

> After the first surgery when I was 17, 18 years old, I had a pessimism about me that almost ruled me. I knew that it wasn't finished, I just knew it. I mean the doctors told me that they took all the disease out, and "You're cured!" and all this stuff. And I remember that day vividly. I just knew that I wasn't finished. . . . There was this monster lingering inside me, and I knew I had to face it once again, and it would be a pretty big battle, and it was.

Such accounts of being pronounced "cured," only to discover that this was rather unlikely in the case of their particular illness, were surprisingly frequent. Thus, the ability of health professionals to accept the chronic condition themselves seemed to play a role in how readily patients and families could accept their situation.

While the informants in this study agreed that acceptance was essential, they varied greatly in their ideas about how to achieve it. For some, it was contingent upon finding answers to their questions about why this unhappy circumstance had befallen them. Such questions often represented theological or moral struggles. For example, one mother of a chronically ill child described agonizing over whether the marijuana she had smoked twice during her pregnancy was the cause of her child's genetic disorder. For many informants, such soul-searching included the experience of either placing blame or deciding that there was nothing and no one to blame. Often, the search for blame seemed to be an essential part of coming to terms with an unexplainable cause. Generally, if families could agree that there was no basis for blame, illness was easier to accept than when they were able to identify a member whose behavior or genetic heritage was at fault.

Talking about the problem was another route to acceptance for many of these patients and families. One woman, for example, explained that acceptance was facilitated by telling friends about the diagnosis. "I'd tell people what it is, and I'd talk, and I'd talk. After a while you can say it without it being painful." Similarly, many of these chronically ill individuals and families reported that they were able to accept their illness only after meeting others who shared the same problem. As one mother recalled, "I had to see another child to believe it, you know, that they look normal and they could read and write and talk and walk, you know, all this kind of thing. But I had to see it for myself."

Several of the informants in this study achieved acceptance by placing their trust in a higher power. One woman, for example, described how such interpretations helped her accept her MS.

> I thought of it as a responsibility to rise to. . . . This meant that it was just a new area that I had never considered becoming part of, that I was going to have a role to play in. . . . For somebody else, that wouldn't work. That would make it more devastating. But, for me, it worked.

Similarly, several patients and families told of paranormal experiences that had facilitated their feeling of acceptance. For example, one mother recalled being visited by an apparition during an intense bout of self-pity.

> He just looked at me, and he looked at [my son], and he smiled and he disappeared. And I've never had anything like that happen to me before. Never! And I just looked at [my son] and I said, "Guess you'll be whatever you're going to be." And I says, "I'll just accept it." And that was it! I just dried up my tears and I've never had another self-pity trip like that. And that's, I figure, when I started accepting him. It was really weird.

While many people were able to accept what had happened to them by drawing on some inner strength supported by beliefs and faith, others needed to rationalize their experience to make sense of it intellectually.

> As time goes by, you rationalize, and you think more logically, you know, well this is the way it is. It cannot change, and it may get better, but basically it's always going to be there. So . . . you must adjust accordingly, and deal with it, and handle it the best way that you can.

For many, this involved placing the illness in the context of other losses that are inherent in being alive, or comparing their chronic illness with a worse one. As one mother remarked, "I'm really grateful. If my kid had to have a catastrophic disease, give me CF." Similarly, patients and families often compared their current health status to the worst case scenario they could anticipate. Through the rational process of considering the very worst possibilities they could imagine, many of these individuals and families found that they could more easily accept the realities of their chronic illness.

For some of those living with chronic illness, acceptance also involved finding some good in an otherwise negative experience. For example, some thought their illness had made them more sensitive and realistic. Others spoke of a heightened appreciation for nature and for the people in their lives. Still others claimed to appreciate the learning brought about by the opportunity to watch themselves change.

> I've done a tremendous amount with the physical side of this being that maybe the writing's on the wall that, okay, it's time to ease off that part, and now we start working a bit more on the emotional and the mental side of that triangle. . . . I feel in transition right now, and not really knowing what I'm going towards.

This new potential for balance and harmony was made possible by recognizing that life included both the good and the bad, and by accepting both as having value.

> I don't know if I can explain it very well at all, but . . . as a result of that experience, I have more of a deeper kind of faith in life and the world, and also a certain baggage of hopelessness that I sometimes sink into. So I don't know exactly what that means, but I'm sort of aware of both instead of just sort of being in a middle kind of place. I feel richer and more powerful sometimes.

Thus, the ability to accept the fact of chronic illness seemed an important component of chronicity for the patients and families in this study. By accepting their circumstances, these men and women freed themselves from questions and doubts, put their experiences into perspective, and found a way to get on with living.

DISCUSSION

In this chapter, the concepts of acuity and chronicity have been used to delineate important aspects of the experience of chronic illness. The accounts paint a portrait of life, including elements inherent in both acuity and chronicity. Their stories provide clear evidence that chronic illness has profound effects upon the emotional, intellectual, social, and instrumental lives of those afflicted (Curtin & Lubkin, 1990). They also illustrate the degree to which the processes of coming to terms with chronic illness and getting on with life are enacted within a social context, and played out on the stage of all of the relationships within the ill person's life (Kasl, 1983).

The notion that chronically ill people experience acute illness and hospitalization differently than do normally well people has been explored in some detail in the scholarly literature. It has been noted that chronically ill patients and their families are indeed perceived as "troublesome" within the health care system by virtue of their greater commitment to controlling their own health care and their heightened capacity to judge the quality of health care work (Thomas, 1987). Thus, the control struggles between the chronically ill and their professional health care providers described in these accounts are far from surprising.

The work involved in chronic illness has been chronicled in detail by Corbin and Strauss (1988). Their description evokes similar images to those generated by the informants in this study, painting a picture of life complicated by medical regimes, time management, and negotiating of health services. This impression of activity, work, and competence strikes an interesting contrast with the more typical social images of victimization and passivity as characteristic of chronicity. Further, the very real social disadvantages, described by these informants as unfriendly physical environments and unsympathetic social services, are also well documented in the literature (Curtin & Lubkin, 1990).

Thus, chronically ill people and their families are thrust into circumstances that require them to engage in considerable analysis and adaptation. While each story is unique, the informants' accounts reveal common themes inherent in chronic illness experience. The accounts make evident the extensive work involved in making sense of the experience, managing emotional responses to the course and prognosis of illness, dealing with acute episodes, and, of course, organizing everyday life. They further reveal the extent to which the social environment, and the health care environment in particular, both help and hinder that work. For the chronically ill, life can be a bitter struggle, a struggle endowed with the potential either to destroy or to enhance quality in living. Understanding the social world in which that struggle is enacted is therefore as important for health professionals and policy-makers as it is for patients and their families.

FOUR

Normalcy and Visibility

In explanations of the social implications of living with chronic illness, the concepts of normalcy and visibility emerged repeatedly. In this chapter, these concepts will be examined in some depth, revealing yet another window from which to view the subjective experience of illness. The frequency with which the chronically ill patients and families referred to an abstract condition called "normal" aroused curiosity about what that notion meant for them. In their accounts, references to normal were intertwined with images of visible and invisible departures from that normal. Thus, accounting for normal requires interpreting what such visible and invisible differences mean in the social world of those who live with chronic illness.

THE MEANING OF NORMAL

The idea of "normal" clearly held meaning for the patients and families in this study and was often cited as a reference point from which to describe their own unique experience. For some, normal meant being able to "fit in." As once patient explained, "I don't want to project an image of invalid, sickly, you know. I want to project an image of well, healthy, able to carry on, able to do things, able to live the normal life." Thus, the ideal of normal included health, but was more strongly linked to the capacity to engage in the activities of everyday living. As one man expressed it, normal meant "not in a healthwise way, but in a lifewise way." Embedded in their use of the concept of normal was an inherent contradiction: that the chronically ill could behave normally but not be normal. One patient's recollections illustrate: "I just carried on as normal as I can, and so people treat me normally. But I'm not." Because they understood normalcy as a social abstraction and an ideal rather than anything tangible, these patients and families began to create complex interpretations of its meaning.

According to many informants, one of the interesting effects of chronic illness was the way it altered one's sense of what was normal. One young diabetic woman, for example, noted that she tended to measure her success in terms of blood glucose levels, while her friends measured theirs in terms of jobs and education. Because effective management of the chronic illness required considerable work, this work eventually became a normal part of living. As one woman explained, "After a while . . . you normalize it."

Their familiarity with illness allowed informants to consider it in the larger context of life events, thereby neutralizing its negative impact. For example, one mother described the following approach to her daughter's illness: "Let's try to deal with it just like you got brown hair and brown eyes, you know, it's part of you. . . . So it's keeping things in perspective. That's normalcy." One man articulated a similar philosophy.

> I look at it this way. I look at a person jogging today, and they look healthy, and who knows, tomorrow they may be hit by a car or something like that. So between the two of us there's not that much difference.

In addition, patients and families talked of putting considerable energy into those aspects of their lives that they considered normal. Many rationalized that their own individual standards, although changed, were consistent with the normal standards for other people, as one man's explanation suggests.

> You've gotta start some place. I guess being satisfied, and content with what you do—even as a carpenter you're used to getting $15, $20 an hour, you know, now your standards have to say, "Hey, $8 an hour's fine, being I'm doing something."

This perspective often included identifying aspects of life in which they were fortunate. No matter how negative the circumstance, there was always a worse case to use as a contrast. As one woman commented, "Even though I may be more crippled, I don't hurt." Another, who did have pain, used the opposite comparison.

> I'll tell you, when I walked down there and saw those young men with only one leg, or one arm, you go back to your room thinking, "What do I have to feel sorry for myself about?" You know, "I'm walking."

Thus, these patients' and families' sense of what was normal evolved through consideration of the problems of others, through inspiration from role models with similar or different health problems, and through placing their illness in the context of other human variations that influence the way that life is lived.

Advantages of Normalizing

By redefining themselves in terms of a modified notion of normalcy, these people were using a strategy which has been referred to in the literature as "normalizing," in which the chronically ill find ways to live as normally as possible despite the symptoms of disease (Knafl & Deatrick, 1986; Strauss et al., 1984). Normalizing helped create a positive attitude toward living with chronic illness, as one woman explained.

> Some people dwell on their illness, and they talk about it all the time, and they get to be a real bore. Well, that doesn't happen here. There's too many interesting things in life to get on with.

In particular, this philosophy appealed to the parents of ill children, for whom normal growth and development was a pressing issue. As one mother commented, "I think you have to understand that these kids are not institutionalized kids. They're kids out in the real world, and they have to be brought up as a normal child."

Many described going to considerable lengths to help their children place the illness in context and feel more normal. One mother recalled reading her child a book about circus freaks to help normalize his physical differences.

> I was showing this to [my son] and talking to him about the people and what they were like personally and what kind of lives they led, you know. A lot of it I'm making up and the rest of it I'm going from just the story line of the book, so that he will grow up with some idea that he's not alone, like this isn't the biggest tragedy in the world.

Thus, for many patients and families, finding ways to feel normal was an important strategy to minimize some of the social effects of having a chronic illness. Toward this end, they attended to the normal aspects of their lives, minimized the significance of any limitations, and appreciated their own circumstances within the context of the wide range of untoward circumstances that could befall people in the course of living.

Disadvantages of Normalizing

In contrast, a number of those living with chronic illness articulated a perspective that departed sharply from such normalization. From their perspective, such a strategy could create serious problems for the individual and family who were faced with a decidedly abnormal situation. For example, some believed that it prevented them from creating a realistic identity, as one woman explained.

> I've always thought of myself as a normal person with maybe this slight little problem (*laugh*) in the background. And I'm beginning to realize that the Myasthenia is very much a part of me, almost like an identity. And it's something I've sort of been denying, which leaves me with absolutely nothing.

Another patient echoed, "I'm not a normal person. I'm not. Unfortunately, that just happens to be the truth."

According to these individuals, trying to normalize caused them to deny the implications of their illness. One young man recalled trying to join his former rugby companions for a celebratory drink after the game. "But now there's no game, you know. You didn't contribute nothing. But you still fake your head off in your mind, to think that, hey, this is just like old times." Thus, the habit of normalizing the illness could have serious long-range implications for such important processes as identity-building and acceptance.

What chronically ill individuals and their families began to realize, they reported, was that "normal" was a largely artificial construct that they, like others in their society, had blindly accepted as valid.

> It's come to me in a great flash of revelation that what's normal for me, is not normal for you. . . . Normal is just a consensus of the majority. That's all it is. It has no meaning. When you really look at it, it has no meaning.

The account of another patient reveals a similar sentiment.

> Normal for me now, after 6 years of TPN (Total Parenteral Nutrition), is what life is on TPN, I guess. I don't try to think of normal as being like everybody else, because that's too hard. . . . So, to me, you know, quote unquote "normal" is just the way of coping the best I can the way I am.

These comments reflected a shared awareness that the notion of normal was a social judgment that valued averageness over individuality. What surprised many of these men and women was the extent to which these assumptions about normalcy had shaped their early adjustment to chronic illness. As one patient recalled, "I was so hooked on normal." Having recognized that the idea of normalcy was one that functionally denied certain aspects of their lives, many patients and families found that they could create a more balanced and whole attitude toward living with chronic illness. Rejecting the social value of normalcy freed them to adopt unique and individualized solutions to the problems they faced.

The accounts portray normalcy as a highly charged concept that has a considerable impact in shaping the way chronically ill people define themselves, manage their lives, and cope with the "abnormalities" of illness. They also reveal normalizing, or redefining the illness to be consistent with normal, to be a double-edged sword, a philosophy that can have beneficial consequences under some circumstances but crippling ones under others. The explanations of normalcy also illustrate the power of the norm in our society as a whole, and suggest some of the values embedded in our tacit assumption that being normal is a decidedly positive attribute.

THE IMPACT OF VISIBLE DIFFERENCES

Among the departures from what is considered normal, visible differences are those that attract our immediate attention and evoke our most spontaneous reactions (Phillips, 1990). In this discussion, the impact of these differences will be considered in the context of social pressure toward normalcy. By examining how the social world responds to a visible difference, and the problems that raises for the people involved, we can arrive at a greater understanding of the interpersonal experience of chronic illness. While the chronically ill do not typically advertise their status to the world at large, certain symptoms or effects of illness make the announcement just as effectively. The most obvious of these are alterations in physical appearance, restrictions in mobility, and unusual behaviors.

Altered Appearance

Many chronic diseases produce some unwelcome alteration to the physical appearance of the ill person. One woman described such changes as a result of arthritis.

I've always loved pretty shoes. I was grieving because my feet were so twisted that I can't wear hardly anything any more. . . . And it changed my speech. It changed my bite . . . so I didn't even look like me any more.

Such changes not only altered how individuals felt about themselves but also forced them to confront the reactions of others. For those whose appearance was significantly altered by chronic illness, being stared at was a major social problem. One mother differentiated friendly from hostile stares. As she explained, "I can accept that, because if he wasn't mine I'd probably do the same. But don't stare at him as if he's a freak and that he ought to have a bullet between his eyes."

Another common situation involved having to respond to questions. For many patients and families, the curiosity of children was easier to accept than was that of adults because it tended to be matter-of-fact and devoid of hidden agendas. As one woman explained, "When kids ask questions, they want just the basics." In fact, many people willingly accepted educating children as a social obligation inherent in having a chronic illness. One mother, for example, allowed her child to be used by an older sibling for "show and tell."

So even if that one handful can come out of that high school being educated, it was well worth taking him up there. At first I wasn't going to, 'cause I thought, I'm not having him as a freak show. And then it dawned on me what could come out of it.

Thus, visible differences in appearance placed chronically ill people and their families in the position of being stared at and being questioned about that difference. For many, this was a nuisance, but an inevitable consequence of living in society. Those who could disguise their altered appearance almost always did so. However, for many, the visible difference was something that profoundly influenced social interaction because of its unrelenting presence.

Restricted Mobility

Limitations in physical mobility represented a related form of visible difference that triggered another set of social responses. Depending on its degree, restricted mobility could be an extremely socially isolating effect of illness. One woman described it as "being like a prisoner." As she said, "My world became the garden and the house." Being mobile was closely linked to normalcy for many informants. For example, one woman preferred suffering pain to being unable to drive because of taking pain killers. "When I'm driving I actually feel normal (*laugh*) because I can drive the car." Similarly, many patients went to considerable effort to remain as mobile as possible for as long as they could.

For many informants, mobility was an essential component of independence. Consequently, compromises to independence were a major source of frustration. Several patients described feeling degraded when forced to ask others for help.

> I don't like to ask anybody . . . for nothing. . . . Maybe it's a sort of pride, and independence, but I don't like to bother people. I like to do my life, and do my business, do my part, and leave me alone. You know. But then you have to change that. You have to start to say, "I'm sorry, I cannot do this, because I got bad legs, I got a heart problem."

Because it threatened their independence, restricted mobility also threatened social credibility, as one woman explained.

> It's the invalidation, that's what it is. A play on words that kept ringing in my mind. There's two ways to pronounce the word i-n-v-a-l-i-d. The invalid is perceived as invalid. Think about it.

According to these people, immobility immediately identified the individual as "disabled," a label which had serious social repercussions. As one woman commented, "I don't want to wear the label 'disabled.' I look at myself—I'm different-abled, that's all." Many recounted personal events as evidence of how society treats its disabled members. For example, one man commented on disabled seating in theaters.

> Now, anywhere along that seating area, there should've been a little cut-out where a wheelchair could park and be up with the rest of the normal people. But no, they don't look at you as a normal person. They put you down there, in this reject area.

One repercussion of being labeled disabled was that even the most well-informed people tended to act nervously in your presence. According to some of these patients and families, it was necessary to devote considerable energy toward putting such people at ease.

> You're the one who shows them how to behave. I mean, some people are made very nervous by your being in a chair, or something. And if you're

sort of cool around them, then they're not nervous around you. So it all depends on your manner, I think.

Because of the awkward responses of those around them, many people with restricted mobility found that social interaction with other disabled individuals was far more satisfying than was coping with the inevitable social reactions among the nondisabled. Despite his early misgivings, one man fondly remembered his first opportunity to spend time with other patients in similar circumstances. "It was active socializing that I could do, and not feel out of place, or a burden to other people, or anything." Like this man, many patients found other disabled people to be accepting of their differences. As one woman said, "Like around a bunch of ordinary folks you might feel that you're unusually klutzy or clumsy. Around them, you're not, which is nice for a change."

Another serious repercussion was the degree to which people were assumed to be mentally incompetent because of a physical disability. As one professional community organizer recalled:

> People would pat me on the head if it came up in conversation anywhere along the line about what I've done, what I want to do on the professional level. People won't accept it, from somebody who's having difficulty walking, that their brain's in place.

The wife of a wheelchair-bound man reported similar frustrations.

> You go in a restaurant and the waitress will come to me and say, "Does he want coffee?" "Ask him!" We've heard this a hundred times! The waitress has asked me right with him 2 feet away, "Do you think he would like to have coffee?" And I say, "Well, ask him." You know, as if he was a complete imbecile.

This anecdote hints at a major irony, according to some of these informants, that having a visible difference actually renders one invisible. One wheelchair-bound man reported that people often completely ignored his greetings when they passed him on the sidewalk. Adding to the intense frustration of such incidents was the knowledge that people generally meant well. For example, one woman recalled an incident in which a friend had come to her home to can strawberries. When it came time to add the pectin, the friend read out the instructions in a painfully slow voice using her finger to point out each word as one might to a child.

A final social effect of the visible mobility impairment, according to the patients and families in this study, is that it conjured up the unrealistic image that ill or disabled individuals are especially virtuous. One woman's explanation of this phenomenon illustrates:

> [A colleague] keeps saying he thinks we're so brave. That is so wrong! I'm sure he feels that, 'cause he thinks, "God, if I ever had that problem I'd never be able to cope that way." And that's not true! Everybody would do—I'm sure everyone would do it the same way. You have to. You do one of two things. You accept it, and cope with it . . . or you kill yourself. . . . You have no choice. It's survival. That's all it is, it's just survival.

From this woman's perspective, the assumption that all disabled people are brave was as unrealistic and patronizing as was the assumption that they were all incompetent. Thus, restricted mobility represented a visible difference that set the chronically ill person apart from the norm, threatened his or her independence, and subjected the individual to a host of demeaning and frustrating social responses.

Unusual Behaviors

Beyond differences in mobility and appearance, several chronically ill individuals and families told of other behaviors that made their illness "visible" in some way. One such behavior described by several individuals was uncontrollable emotional lability. For example, tearfulness at inappropriate times could be a highly noticeable difference, as one woman explained:

> When you're visiting with someone, all of a sudden you start crying—there is some little thing I've said, or they've said—and then you feel like a donkey 'cause you can't say exactly why you're crying.

One woman reported having to give up tutoring because of changes to her voice, another social visible difference. "The poor kids would think I was drunk, or something. I mean, I sound drunk to some people, although I'm not. I don't drink. But my speech gets screwy."

For those patients and families in whom chronic illness required dietary alterations, the visibility of eating became quite apparent. As one man explained, "An intestinal disease affects you so profoundly, because food is the basis of social things." Others talked of making people nervous by not eating, or by eating noticeably different diets at family celebrations and other occasions. For such individuals, the social pressures surrounding food consumption were particularly conspicuous.

Other unusual behaviors described by some of these patients and families included such symptoms as noxious odors, audible bowel sounds, or flatulence. While not visible in the usual sense, such phenomena could be difficult to disguise and made the illness dramatically evident to others, as one woman's comments illustrate.

> It's a disease that is extremely isolating, mostly because of the smell that's associated with Crohn's. It's very offensive. And all the time going to the can. The bowel movements are usually quite offensive, even if it's mostly liquid. There's also a tremendous amount of gas, which is also very offensive. This is very isolating for people who are shy, who are timid, who don't know how to deal with this, who don't know anybody who can say, "Look, I fart a lot now, and it's pretty awful!" They've got to try and get up and run out on the room if they've got guests, or they can't go to a concert. It becomes a very isolating, and a very lonely disease.

According to the men and women involved, such symptoms violated social taboos, creating an immediate social strain. Most patients with such problems preferred voluntary isolation to dealing with the difficult social repercussions. In contrast, however, some informants became skilled at making normally unmentionable bodily functions socially acceptable to those around them. One woman described her matter-of-fact approach to self-catheterizing her urinary bladder this way.

> I'm so up-front about my "job," as I call it. That was the best way with the children, because when they're here, Grandma has to go and do her job in the bedroom, and I shut the door, and they want to know why they can't come in. So it's Grandma's job time, and you wait till Grandma's through, and then you can see Grandma.

A final difference that was reported by several informants was forgetfulness, which could also generate extremes in social discomfort. One woman reported that a common response to her forgetfulness was to minimize its importance. She observed, "Like so many people say, 'Well, I don't remember things either.' It isn't the same, you know." From her perspective, attempts to normalize this extremely frustrating symptom were quite patronizing. Thus, according to these ill individuals and families, evidence of unusual behaviors could set apart the ill person in much the same way as did altered appearance and restricted mobility.

Implications of Visible Difference

By making chronic illness visible, such differences brought it into the social arena, where it was then the target for a variety of responses. In some instances, there were advantages to having a visible difference. According to one patient, being visibly different afforded you the opportunity of creating a sympathetic community.

> When there is some, you know, incapacity, or some crippling, or something visual, then, of course, people are more able to identify with that, and ask questions, or feel sorry for you, or know there's something not quite right about you.

At times, the visible difference legitimized certain forms of assistance. For example, one woman found supermarket attendants much more likely to assist her with heavy groceries when she was wearing her cervical collar.

However, according to most patients and families, the advantages were outweighed by the frustrating and demoralizing social implications inherent in being easily identifiable. The visible difference meant that they were no longer dealt with as an individual but were stereotyped as disabled. As one informant complained, "I don't like people who talk to me like I'm a disease." Being included in generalizations rather than identified as a unique individual was therefore a particularly frustrating social implication of a visible difference for many of those living with chronic illness.

A related but even more disturbing repercussion of having a visible difference was that it created the real possibility of discrimination. While actual episodes of discrimination were not frequently reported among these informants, there was agreement that a visible difference made one especially vulnerable to them. Jean and Bill, for example, were taken to court following a vehicular accident because the driver of the other car assumed that Bill's obvious handicap would place him at fault.

The chronically ill individuals and families in this study, therefore, described the social effects of a visible difference as frustrating, demeaning, demoralizing, and invalidating. By virtue of a visible difference, they became subject to the effects of intolerance and ignorance in their social universe. In many cases, they formed theories as to why people behaved as insensitively and as rudely as they did and developed creative strategies to cope with the social reverberations they could not avoid.

Within the social worlds of the patients and families, however, the intolerance and ignorance of one particular group of people was most difficult to rationalize and to accept. The accounts of these people suggested that health care professionals demonstrated similar prejudices toward visible differences as did less-informed members of society. For example, one family recalled a doctor avoiding their child with CP.

> When we first moved down here I would take [my son] in for an ear infection, for example, [the doctor] would stand at the other side of the room and kind of look at [him] like this, "Oh, he looks fine to me." You know, as if he's going to catch the disease. And that's not exaggerating. It was just terrible!

When health care professionals responded in ways that revealed no sympathy with or understanding of visible differences, these ill individuals and families felt especially betrayed, as one man noted. "There are so many diseases that incapacitate you, that when a nurse or health care worker or anybody sees it, they automatically associate it with a mental incapacitation also. That's really annoying for me." Another individual told a story that illustrated the display of similar attitudes toward her ill husband.

> I went and talked with the doctor after [my husband] had come out, and he said, "Well, I'm prescribing this for him." I said, "Okay." And he said, "You know, he's actually quite smart. He's really got himself together." And I just looked at him and said, "Well, of course he's smart. There's nothing wrong with his brain" (*laugh*). I mean, since he saw someone in a wheelchair, you know, it was obvious to me he classified everyone in a wheelchair as like the people sitting in the old folks' home over there, you know. And it was almost like he was surprised.

While patients and families were astonished by such ignorance among health care professionals, they were also horrified at the thought that such attitudes might influence treatment recommendations. For example, one mother recalled such an instance. When her child was sent home on a powerful anticoagulant medication, the doctor failed to recommend a safety helmet, assuming that the mother's preference would be to have her child "look normal." Discovering that the helmet was standard practice for "normal" children on that drug, she was convinced that her child's safety had been jeopardized by prejudice.

Thus, the accounts of the patients and families in this study illustrate extreme social pressure to conform to an ideal of "normal" and, if they cannot, to accept the consequent social distance their illness creates. Their accounts make it evident that having a difference is often far less consequential than is being seen to have a difference. In this way, they further illustrate how deeply grounded the experience of chronic illness is in a social context.

THE IMPACT OF INVISIBLE DIFFERENCES

Among the many possible effects of chronic illness, there are those that are socially invisible (Alonzo, 1985). According to the patients and families in this study, the experience of invisible differences is far more complex than simply that of avoiding the problems of visibility. The most common invisible differences that these men and women talked about were fatigue and pain. A description of the accounts of what it is like to live with these particular problems will therefore illuminate yet another set of reactions that make up the social experience of chronic illness.

Fatigue

Among the invisible symptoms of illness that patients and families described, fatigue was the most common and often most debilitating. While fatigue has long been recognized as an effect of illness, it is typically interpreted as a relatively minor inconvenience. However, for many of these people, fatigue was of such an extreme degree that it bore little relationship to the phenomenon that well people call by the same name, as one woman's description illustrates:

> There's tired, and there's MS tired. It's two totally different things, you know. Most people are tired, and a good night's sleep'll do it. We're talking tired here to die, right? Tired, where someone screamed, "Fire," and the building was in flames, and you'd say, "Well, I'm just too damn tired," you know . . . too tired to pick up your toothbrush . . . you're hungry, you're thirsty, whatever, too tired to go into the kitchen. That's tired.

Because it was an invisible symptom, such intense fatigue was impossible for others to fully appreciate. Further, because it prevented people from performing certain expected functions, their fatigue exposed them to criticism. One young MS patient recalled being considered a "lazy fool" in high school because of her inability to participate in physical education.

While fatigue also affected their emotional state, most informants believed that deliberately understating their fatigue was a critical social strategy, as one woman's experience illustrates:

> Phony as it might be . . . I simply can't imagine in all those years my husband coming home to somebody who was not cheerful. . . . So there again there was a lot of suppression going on, but I felt it was essential.

Thus, fatigue was a common invisible difference that evoked a critical social response, requiring some pretense in its management. Because people with fatigue did not behave normally, yet had no visible excuses for their lack of participation, they were required to cover up or face social condemnation.

Pain

Unlike fatigue, pain is something for which people tend to have a great deal of sympathy. However, such sympathy is generally reserved for those circumstances in which we believe pain to be severe, such as childbirth, multiple trauma, or end-stage cancer. It is far more difficult to identify with chronic pain, partly because the individual does not exhibit those characteristics we associate with "true" pain, such as screaming, grimacing, crying, or muscle rigidity. When people can apparently walk, talk, and function normally, our ability to appreciate their pain seems greatly diminished (Lubkin, 1990a).

According to the accounts of the patients and families in this study, chronic pain had a profound influence on their ability to participate in and enjoy life. Because their pain was invisible to others, these men and women often suffered silently. As one woman ruefully noted, "I guess if I had a cast on my arm people would say, 'That's too bad, it must be painful.' " However, it took a considerable amount of work to behave normally when in pain, as one patient noted: "You're aware of trying to combat the pain and be cheerful . . . to not let it get the best of you. . . . So it takes extra energy to keep smiling."

For most people, it was important to learn to avoid complaining about their pain. One woman remarked, "If one were to always complain about it, you'd be complaining all the time." As one man noted, it was difficult to convey essential information about the implications of his pain without appearing to complain.

> I would always downplay it. Just say, "My back's a little sore." But they should know that that means that they should do the dishes (*laugh*), or they should do something, (*laugh*) you know, without me having to bitch and complain about it.

Another challenge had to do with deciding when and with whom to be honest about the pain. A double bind for many of these people was that they needed to communicate about the pain in order to be understood, but were hesitant to say too much for fear of being discounted. While self-protection was critical for many individuals in pain, they courted social rejection because of their unwillingness to perform certain expected actions, as one man with chronic back pain recalled:

> Sometimes I'm in a certain situation, and people look to me to do the lifting. And if you're in a room with three women and a child, and something needs lifting, everybody looks to you. . . . But it bugs me that they think that, you know. They look at me, and my physical appearance is pretty healthy, like I'm not fat or nothing, so they think, "Why can't he do it?" That bugs me.

Thus pain, like fatigue, created an invisible yet real departure from normalcy for these patients. For this reason, several people found that chronic pain led them to seek socialization with those most likely to understand it. One young woman explained shifting to a social group that was senior to her by a generation in order to find support.

> Some of your younger friends, they can't relate, which is understandable, to a degree, and then they don't realize what you're going through at all. Whereas some of those older people do. So maybe I get along with people who have been through pain.

According to these patients and families, chronic pain was a significant factor in their emotions, in their ability to enjoy life, and in their physical performance. By explaining their pain to others, they risked being considered overly self-centered; however, by trying to appear normal, they risked being considered lazy, inconsiderate, or boring. Therefore, many altered their social patterns in some way to avoid this bind, seeking relationships in which empathy was more likely or circumstances in which their performance was less likely to be judged lacking.

Implications of Invisible Differences

To some extent, these chronically ill individuals and families recognized that there could be advantages in invisibility, in that it allowed for a "semblance of normalcy." For example, where those with visible differences had no choice in the message they communicated to the world at large, those with invisible symptoms did have choices. When such symptoms were manageable, invisibility afforded the patient the option of appearing normal.

In contrast, the patients and families clearly articulated a number of serious disadvantages to having an invisible difference. The most common and often the most distressing of these was that they had trouble convincing others that their illness was legitimate. As one man recalled, "Lots of times people would just [think], 'Aren't you kind of overdoing . . . or playing this up a little bit?' " When their observations did not conform to expectations of what an ill person should look like, people tended to become intolerant and to suspect that the individual with invisible differences was exaggerating the effects of illness. Several informants described situations in which they had been criticized, overtly or covertly, because their illness was not legitimized by their overt appearance.

> If you look okay and you still don't do things, like you don't get all the dishes done, or the housework done, or your papers written, or everything—first-class—and you look all right, then it has to be here (*points to head*), you know. Or you're lazy. All those pejorative terms come out. We're often only given credence or legitimacy for not doing things by having something very observable.

According to several of the informants, this social value derived from the traditional assumption that hard work and perseverance solve all ills. Thus, in addition to the direct effects of the illness itself, the experience of these informants included some rather painful criticisms from those around them.

While not all of these informants experienced such disapproval, they all agreed that invisible symptoms made empathy from others difficult.

As one man discovered, "The only ones that would come close were maybe somebody with the same kind of illness or chronic condition. They would understand." Another way in which invisible differences disadvantaged these patients was that they failed to provide the sorts of cues by which people remembered to account for limitations. Thus, the invisibility of their differences sometimes placed patients in situations of misunderstanding which could be frustrating, isolating, or even threatening to their health.

Because they exercised some freedom over the extent to which they made their illness public, some of these people also suffered the effects of having tried to pass for normal. For example, passing for normal denied them the opportunity to be credited for accomplishments while ill, as one patient recalled:

> In all those years when I was truly ill, I disguised it as much as possible. I didn't want people to know what was wrong with me and I hid it. . . . And I wish I could say, "Hey, listen, I've been through a lot and I'm the best I can be, and don't make out that I'm not capable enough, because I'm really doing well." But you can't say that. . . . There is no room for those concessions.

When others were unaware of the illness, there was an increased risk of acutely uncomfortable social encounters. For example, one family described a painful episode that occurred when their 12-year-old daughter, who had CF, insisted that the parents not inform her new teacher of the illness. One day, the teacher showed the class a film in which CF was described as a fatal disease, a description that the daughter had not heard to this point. Further, people worried about the social embarrassment inherent in being caught passing for normal. According to one man, such discovery was inevitable. "If you're phony about it you're going to suffer." Thus, trying to pass for normal was an option for those with some invisible differences, but an option that created a new set of hazards.

The accounts of invisible differences clearly illustrate the social disadvantages involved. According to these patients and families, differences that are not visible provoke incredulous reactions in others, invalidating the seriousness of the disease itself or ascribing negative personality qualities to the individual afflicted. Invisible differences make empathy difficult and therefore create tensions between those with such symptoms and those without. Furthermore, attempting to pass for normal raises its own set of problems. It seems that there are few socially appropriate ways in which an invisible difference can be effectively communicated.

Clearly, the social world in which people experience invisible differences shapes many aspects of their overall experience. The responses and attitudes of others create a climate that discredits the person whose illness cannot be legitimized visually. The accounts reflect the emotional distress that such discrediting precipitated. Many people with invisible differences, like those with visible differences, experienced a social world which was intolerant and unsympathetic. Further, they also found that such attitudes extended even to those individuals who should have been better informed—the professional health care providers.

According to these patients and families, it was especially frustrating to have professionals doubt their discomfort simply because they could not see it. As one man noted, "You feel defensive, as if you have to prove there's something wrong."

The informants found that, when refined assessment methods and technological instruments were insufficient to measure the illness, the professionals responded the same way as did the general public to lack of visual confirmation. For example, one woman recalled a frustrating incident in which she was not believed until the doctor finally saw the symptom first-hand.

> I was irate, and I said I didn't want to be told it was in my head. I wanted to be examined properly, and to find out what was going on. And he asked me could I show him a spasm in my legs. And I said, "Well, I don't really know . . . I'll try." And I was sitting in the chair, and I just moved my leg up and down, from the knee, just sort of like that, to see what would happen. And it went into spasm. And he held it while it just shook. . . . He sort of patted me nicely, and he said, "Well . . . yes, you do have them, don't you? They are real." And he went through the whole process of sort of reassuring me nicely but in a rather paternal way.

Further, these informants were often perturbed to discover that health care professionals relied heavily on superficial visual cues to assess what life was really like for the patient, as one woman's remarks illustrate:

> Every time he comes in here he says, "You look good." I said, "Doctor, don't you say that to me again." I hate it when people say, "But you look so well." I feel fine, it's just that I can't walk, which is very frustrating.

While these patients and families could understand the ignorance of lay people with regard to the relationship between appearance and illness, they were rather horrified when it occurred among those who ought to know better, as one account illustrates:

> [The doctor] also said to me, "I've never had a scleroderma patient before." Well, many doctors never have. So he said, "The only one I saw was in hospital when I was taking my training." And he said, "You don't look anything like her. You must be very mild." And I thought that that's so ignorant because a doctor should know that there's no two scleroderma cases alike. Each person is hit differently, and some of my friends with scleroderma who are very ill look the picture of health. There is so much wrong inside of them you can see in their eyes if you look. . . . So here's this doctor saying that I must be very mild because of my appearance, and he of all people should know that with scleroderma you can't go by appearance.

In some cases, such disbelief or misinterpretation resulted in professionals judging patients to be undeserving of certain services. For example, one young woman with severe muscle weakness discovered that the occupational therapist was unwilling to order a special nail clipper. "She has things that would help me to access a, quotation marks, 'normal life-style,' and she's telling me that it's for people who are more abnormal than me!" Another patient, whose doctor had strongly recommended increasing her home support services, was turned down because the seriousness of her illness was invisible to the home support investigator.

> Now I was dressed, you know, my hair was done and my make-up. I like to look nice. . . . So she saw what I looked like and made her decision on that instead of going any further. . . . I cut off my nose to spite my face. I refused to really lay it out and beg and plead, you know, make it look bad. . . . It's funny. But even though I knew she was coming I still put my make-up on, you know.

According to these patients and families, many health care professionals required visual confirmation of the illness before they were comfortable offering help. One patient attributed his difficulty obtaining adequate pain relief in the hospital to his generally healthy appearance. Another theorized that such professionals need patients to assume the expected dependent status.

I find this very often, that if you're in control of yourself, if you have your dignity about you, you're not heard. But if you can pull the plug and fall apart at the seams, it's almost as if the person at the other end—the medical support system, or whatever—has to feel in the driver's seat and say, "I know what I can do for you. Here, look, we can help you out this way." They don't like being asked for help, they like offering help.

Thus, invisible differences eroded the credibility of chronically ill individuals and often prevented them from obtaining necessary services. From the point of view of these patients and families, the absence of visual confirmation of the disease thereby created a serious impediment to obtaining health care.

DISCUSSION

The accounts of these informants portray a tangled and complex social world in which chronic illness is defined, interpreted, and judged. In so doing, they illustrate the extent to which chronic illness is a product of social construction. From a sociological point of view, people are sick when they act sick (Cole & Lejeune, 1987). In chronic illness, there are considerable variations both in whether one wants to act sick and in how one goes about enacting that option if one so chooses (Alonzo, 1985).

The accounts make evident the extent to which an abstract notion of what is normal becomes the standard against which much of life is measured by and for the chronically ill. In the social science literature, the idea of normal as an inherent standard of functioning has been examined in some detail. According to Wright (1982), we tend to judge health in terms of the individual's ability to perform in normal social situations, thereby ascribing both social and moral qualities to the concept. Armstrong (1983) explains that, while the term *normal* in the statistical sense refers to a usual measure or tendency, its social definition equates it to such attributes as acceptability and desirability. When people redefine their own standard of normal on the basis of their own everyday life experience, they include a greater range of humanity in the equation and modify the criteria by which social desirability is to be judged. Thus, a standard of normality becomes individualized (Calnan, 1987).

The advantages of normalizing as a basic strategy of social and health care policy have received considerable scholarly attention. As a strategy, it charges society with providing the resources and conditions under which the ill or handicapped may create as normal a life as is possible for them (Wolfensberger, 1980a). The underlying philosophy is clearly motivated by humanitarian objectives, including the perceived right of individuals "not to be different" (Wolfensberger, 1980b). As such, it has received widespread acceptance within the health care community (Wood-Dauphinee & Williams, 1987).

However, according to the accounts of the informants in this study, an emphasis on normalizing may disadvantage some individuals with chronic illness. Strauss and colleagues (1984) acknowledge that such normalizing can require ingenuity and hard work in the extreme. Further, there is no real evidence that this effort results in increased life satisfaction (Cameron, Titus, Kostin, & Kostin, 1973). From the informants' perspective, normalizing can represent a subtle but penetrating form of denial. While the literature differentiates normalizing from denial according to whether the illness is "acknowledged" (Knafl & Deatrick, 1986), this criterion seems an artificial one in the context of the rich accounts of the complexities of acceptance articulated here. Thus, such a perspective may reveal more about the discomfort health professionals have in facing these unpalatable realities than it articulates a genuinely useful distinction. Murphy, Scheer, Murphy, and Mack (1988) point out that what health care professionals consider "acceptance" might be more accurately described as passive endorsement of services. However, the power of the social standard called "normal" is evident in these accounts. Further, the informants in this study illustrate how this standard can be manipulated to their advantage under certain circumstances, and can create new sets of problems under others.

The degree to which the manifestations of illness are visible has also been depicted as an important variable in the social experience of living with chronic illness. Visible signs mark the ill person as different, thereby subjecting him or her to negative stereotypes and possible discrimination (O'Neill, 1985). According to the oral narratives gathered by one author, popular American culture depicts those with visible disabilities as "damaged goods" (Phillips, 1990). Through a process called "identity spread," visible differences are generalized to include other perceived incapacities, such as mental incompetence or deafness (Strauss et al., 1984). In addition, the stigma associated with disease creates conditions under which discrediting the ill person is socially sanctioned (Scambler, 1984). The accounts of the informants in this study illustrate each of these processes in action.

In contrast to people with many other stigmatizing conditions, such as racial or religious minorities, the visibly disabled are not taught how to manage discrediting through the mechanisms of socialization within the family (Murphy et al., 1988). Rather, they are generally left to make sense of it on their own. According to Zola (1982), the absence of formal learning opportunities can result in the adoption of rather unrealistic role models, such as elite athletes, as the standard of what the disabled are expected to achieve. Thus, the societal trend toward normalizing creates conditions in which the visibly disabled are challenged by impractical ideals and, at the same time, discredited for what they are able to accomplish.

The individual whose illness is invisible may have more options as to how his or her condition will be socially portrayed. However, according to these informants, there are important ways in which invisibility also creates disadvantages. The social science literature again offers some explanations. It has been noted that in the absence of visible signs of illness, the individual is generally subjected to the expectations placed upon healthy individuals (Stephenson & Murphy, 1986). In order to be exempt from such behavioral expectations, a complex combination of excuses, disclaimers, and justifications becomes the means by which the illness is socially negotiated (Alonzo, 1985). In the case of certain conditions whose diagnosis is imprecise, problems with establishing legitimacy also extend into the health care context (Strauss et al., 1984). However, legitimizing the illness invariably spoils normal identity (Morgan et al., 1985). Thus, chronic illness becomes a situation in which you are "damned if you do and damned if you don't." As Zola explains, "In trying to plan our lives, we are either pushed to regard our physical difficulty as the all-encompassing touchstone or to claim that we are just like everyone else, needing or wanting no special consideration" (1982, p. 230).

In the case of both visible and invisible differences, then, departures from normal are judged negatively and treated harshly. According to Zola, the social world of the chronically ill is characterized by two major concepts: infantilization and invalidation (1982, p. 235). The informants in this study have articulated such experiences vividly. Further, they have told us that such experiences extend into the arena of professional health care. According to Livneh (1984), the origins of these negative attitudes toward the disabled run deep within the very fabric of our society, thus are not amenable to rapid change. However, those patients and families who are living with chronic illness have obviously been forced to revise their own attitudes and, therefore, have little patience with the intolerance and indignity they suffer at the hands of those who are resistant to attitudinal change. From the perspective of the chronically ill and their families, such resistance within the health care system is all the more frustrating and infuriating because it seems entirely inexcusable.

PART TWO

The Interpersonal Experience

Relationships With Health Care Providers

The previous chapters have provided a graphic description of ways in which chronic illness is experienced by those individuals and families involved. Listening to the stories of the onset and diagnosis of a chronic illness, we have heard how important health care professional competence and consideration were for patients and families. Interpreting what chronicity entails in everyday life, and how acute illness disrupts its tentative balance, we have understood the immense gulf between how people with chronic illness live and how people within their social and health care worlds expect them to live. Finally, by exploring what the chronically ill have to tell us about their sense of normalcy and their experience with visible and invisible differences, we have come to appreciate the social climate within which the chronically ill must carve their new roles and identities. Further, we have learned that the professional health care arena is neither a refuge from this unwelcome social climate nor a reliable source of support in helping chronically ill people deal with a largely unsympathetic and intolerant world.

In this chapter, our consideration of the experience of chronic illness will shift its focus toward a direct examination of those health care relationships in which the chronically ill negotiate their illnesses and create the strategies that will shape their futures. The accounts in the previous chapters have alluded to the significance of health care relationships in many aspects of the complex and demanding process of acquiring and living with a chronic illness. Health care professionals clearly hold the weight of authority in judging the merits of people's health complaints, determining a diagnosis and a course of treatment, and controlling access to precious health-related resources. Their actions and attitudes play an enormous part in determining the degree of distress that patients and families will have in the course of their chronic illness experience. Therefore, what these people have to tell us about health care relationships will raise to a higher level our understanding of why chronic illness is experienced as it is in our society.

THE SIGNIFICANCE OF HEALTH CARE RELATIONSHIPS

The accounts of the chronically ill individuals and families in this study confirmed that the caliber of health care relationships is central to the quality of health care and to the experience of living with a chronic illness. They made explicit how such relationships make a significant difference, in either a positive or a negative direction, to all facets of life for the chronically ill and their families.

While this study concerned itself with health care relationships of all stripes, the accounts made it evident that the physician was most often the pivotal figure from the patient's and the family's perspective. Because physicians were generally in positions of decision-making authority, because they were the first point of contact for many patients, and because they were regarded as senior members of the health care team, physicians were most often named in the accounts. However, because the illness experience led them through a variety of health care settings and services, most patients and families had some involvement with a great many professionals of other persuasions. The attention in this discussion will focus on health care encounters that were sufficiently enduring to permit a relationship to develop between provider and recipient. As will be explained in later chapters, the professionals with whom the encounter was brief tended to become extensions of the system itself in the minds of the individuals and families with chronic illness. In contrast, the professionals most intimately involved in the ongoing management of chronic illness entered relationships which, for their patients, quickly became as significant as any in their lives.

According to these informants, an ongoing relationship with a health care professional was especially important in chronic illness. As one man commented, "Doctors that don't look after you regularly don't . . . give you the same feeling of confidence as your long-term doctor." Often, the primary value of such long-term relationships was having someone to talk to. For example, one woman reflected on the importance of her nurse clinician, saying, "I couldn't have survived if I couldn't have phoned her and talked to her." As another patient explained, health care relationships could provide the validation essential in chronic illness. "Sometimes you don't even need problem solving, you just need to have somebody hear you and understand." When patients and family members found relationships that met their needs in this regard, they became quite committed to them, as one woman's account illustrates.

> You know, I think one of the greatest of fears in many of the people at the clinic, of the parents, is that [the nurse]'s going to leave her job one day . . . and I don't like that. . . . I mean [that nurse] knew my kid had CF before I knew my kid had CF, you know. She was hours ahead of me on knowing it, and she has much more understanding, you know. So I rely on her expertise—about, you know, what it's all about and the liaison between her and the doctors, you know. Because the doctors are okay, but they're not as good.

While these chronically ill individuals and families genuinely welcomed ongoing relationships in health care, they were acutely aware of the way that a professional role circumscribed the boundaries of such associations. As one patient explained, "They can't be socially interested." In addition, they seemed highly attuned to variations in the role requirements of the various professions. "I think doctors like to keep their distance from the patients. The nurses are more like friends of yours." Thus, they agreed that health care relationships made a vital contribution to the experience of living with chronic illness.

THE PROCESS OF HEALTH CARE RELATIONSHIP EVOLUTION

The accounts of these patients and families revealed that relationships between them and their health care providers were dynamic and had evolved over time. From their perspective, the process of health care relationships in chronic illness seemed to involve predictable shifts in attitudes, emotions, and behaviors (Thorne & Robinson, 1988a). These shifts were characterized by discoveries and insights that helped the chronically ill person and family make sense of the experience in which they found themselves. As one informant noted, "It's like a turnaround, and you have to break a lot of patterns . . . a lot of thought patterns . . . a lot of old habits." Although involvement with health care professionals was hardly a new experience for people, chronic illness reframed such health care relationships into a new and different context.

Patients and families explained the process of health care relationships in terms of recognizing and confronting the differences created by chronic illness. As one man described it, "At different stages, depending on what's happening, you know, you go through great feelings of anger or frustration. . . . You maybe subconsciously sort of sit back and take some stock-taking, so to speak." Analysis of the data revealed three distinct stages through which these health care relationships progressed: naive trust, disenchantment, and guarded alliance.

Naive Trust

When they looked back on the beliefs and attitudes they had held at the outset of the health care relationships, patients and their families realized that they had operated under the illusion that the health care professional would understand the nature of the problem and would find a solution to it. They recalled that they entered their early health care relationships with the assumption that the professional would know what was in the best interests of the patient and family and, further, would initiate whatever was necessary to facilitate those best interests. They remembered believing that health care professionals were omnipotent and altruistic, capable of solving all manner of health problems. One woman recalled, "At first, I guess like most people . . . I just saw doctors as being, you know—I put them on a pedestal." By placing their faith in the experts, these chronically ill individuals and their families anticipated that they would be guided through the process of obtaining health care in whatever form was best suited to their needs.

In light of these beliefs, patients and families claimed that they were passive and expectant in this initial stage of the health care relationship. As one woman explained, "I was very much in the child role almost at that time, I would say, because I was just putting myself into their hands and trusting as a child is." Thus, they placed themselves under the complete control of the health professionals and obediently waited for the answer to their problem. This passive stance meant that they expected to be involved in decisions about the health care problem only if and when the professional asked for their input. Thus, in many cases, it did not occur to them to make suggestions or even to ask questions. As one patient recalled, "I never thought to ask for physio. I figured if

I really needed it, the doctor would tell me." Another described a similar perspective.

> At the beginning I had an attitude that because they were health care professionals, they would have the answers and that whatever they said, or whatever their decisions were, would be more knowledgeable than what I would think or what my decisions would be.

Further, these chronically ill individuals and families anticipated that any decisions made on their behalf probably reflected a genuine concern on the part of the professional to provide whatever was best in their particular case. Therefore, as one patient remembered, they were inclined to go along with all recommendations. As one patient recalled, "When I was diagnosed, Dr. M., the internist, said, 'There's no point in treating you if you don't quit smoking.' So I quit smoking. . . . If he said quit breathing, I'd quit!"

While the patients and families recalled rather vague and unrealistic expectations of what would happen to them in the context of their health care relationships, they remembered being certain that if they trusted their health professional completely, all would be well. As one man commented, "I used to believe that a doctor was like a god. When you walked into a doctor's office, if he said something, that was it." A young woman's depiction of her parents' attitudes graphically illustrates such absolute faith. "[My parents] hung on a doctor's every word, you know. Like if a doctor said, 'Go out and eat these snails, rub oil on your belly every time, and you'll be 20 years younger,' they would have done it!" As another informant explained, at this stage she would have jumped off a bridge had her doctor so recommended.

In this initial stage of the health care relationship, patients and families recalled believing that complete trust was necessary to secure healing and facilitate the helping process. Thus, they explained their initial attitude toward the health care relationship as a naive trust that those in whom they had invested authority over their well-being actually possessed the necessary knowledge and mercy. As one man explained, "You give yourself into their hands to take care of you and make you whole. I mean it's almost a quasi-religious experience!"

When they later looked back on this early stage, these patients and families were often incredulous about the extent of their naiveté and the unequivocal nature of their trust.

I realize now that I was a very sick individual, and at that time I had really given up a lot of my power and placed it in the hands of the medical professionals, and they in fact were really controlling this illness, or the supposed direction of this illness.

Thus, the stage of naive trust was one in which expectations were high, trust was absolute, and people tended to be confident that their health care professionals would help them solve their health care problems, whatever they turned out to be.

Disenchantment

Inevitably, the course of events made such an uninformed and trusting stance untenable. In some cases, the naive trust was shattered early on in the chronic illness, as one informant recalled.

You go in with the doctors and the nursing profession on a pedestal. You really do! You think that they're so knowledgeable and so caring, and they know so much, and that everything they say is gospel. But you soon find out it isn't! That was the biggest shock.

In other cases, the trust endured for some time into the experience. For most patients and families, naive trust was sufficiently ingrained that it remained intact until major difficulties forced them to rethink it, as one man explained.

Those that are brought up to believe in that system . . . the medical system . . . stay with it until they reach a point of total frustration, or there's no resolution to their problem, before they start seeking alternatives.

For some of those living with chronic illness, the transition out of naive trust was triggered by a single event of such proportion that trust was out of the question. One woman, for example, explained that her trust was shattered when her physician reneged on his agreement to change the treatment plan, without offering a viable rationale.

So I went through all this rigmarole of having [the diagnostic procedure] done, and when they got the results back and everything was looking good he says, "Well, it's looking good but I still think we'll keep you on [the medication]." And I was furious at him, and then I thought . . . well, I knew I would never go back to that doctor. And I really started to question then, too.

Another found trust impossible to sustain when her doctor failed to visit her during a hospitalization. She said, "Can you imagine being in there for a month, and never seeing your doctor, not even once?" A third patient attributed his shattered trust to the realization that his doctor was unable to acknowledge the benefits of his health promotion efforts.

> I started taking vitamins to get rid of my cold, and the doctor told me I was pissing my money away. And so I left him, because I knew that the vitamins had helped me . . . I wasn't getting any colds. He said, "I haven't seen you for months. Why haven't you come for . . . " you know, and I said, "It's because I've been taking vitamins." And that was his response. So I said, "Well, to hell with you. I'm going to find another doctor who listens to me."

For other patients and families, no single episode accounted for the transition; rather, a series of events or experiences gradually began to shake the foundations of the trust. One woman expressed the process this way: "Each time something happens . . . you seem to shrink a little bit more." Thus, the loss of trust was often the culmination of a number of events that eroded people's confidence and caused them to rethink their experience.

While events triggering the transition were various and individual, some common themes emerged from the accounts. One such theme was the perception that information was being withheld from the patient and family. Another was that the overall objectives of the professionals were often radically different from those of the chronically ill individuals and families. A third source of difficulty arose from the realization that health care professionals were more concerned with their careers than they were with the actual care and support of their patients. As one individual angrily pointed out, "I have seen and felt that we were being used—that we were just things." Events of this nature forced these patients and families to confront their unmet expectations to the extent that they could no longer excuse or explain them according to their old beliefs.

The transition into the second stage, disenchantment, was a time of utter frustration and intense self-doubt for these chronically ill individuals and families. In the form of a harsh and shocking realization, they began to understand that the anticipated help would not be provided for them in the way that they had expected. As one man said, "It frustrates you to no end to realize that you're not going to get any help from anybody." While their naive trust had been a source of comfort and stability in the early stages of illness, the shattering of this trust set them adrift in a sea of anxiety and fear, frustration and anger, insecurity and self-doubt. As one patient recalled, "I was left hanging, totally left hanging."

The informants portrayed themselves as being vulnerable, confused, and quite out of control during the stage of disenchantment. As one mother of a chronically ill child complained, "It's like we're all puppets." Another woman described her experience with a similar tone of frustration.

> They just pat you on the knee, you have this thing that you can't pronounce, and then you have to go from there. "Don't worry Mrs. X., we'll get you a wheelchair when you need one." This is what I was left with!

According to these patients and families, the stage of disenchantment was an emotional and cognitive nightmare. They recalled acting out their intense frustrations in the form of aggressive and hostile behaviors, often directed toward the health care professionals. One woman relayed the following episode: "I went up to the [nursing] station and screamed and ranted and raved. . . . I made a huge scene, actually." Another recalled a similar reaction: "I think when I was really angry at the system, I got incredibly mouthy about it and quite verbal. I was quite nasty in some of my comments."

The patients and families explained these behaviors as their reaction to shattered trust. Frequently, they reported questioning the wisdom of these aggressive responses even as they were engaged in them. Many men and women described such acting-out behaviors as counterproductive to both their health care relationships and their ability to obtain health care service. They also reported feeling acutely anxious about the potential repercussions of these acting-out behaviors. Generally, they expected or actually experienced some sort of retaliation on the part of the health care professionals. One mother of an ill child explained why she thought such retaliation was likely.

> I think that's a situation that certainly if I was a nurse I would have a feeling I would fall prey to—that, you know, that if the mother drove me crazy I would have a tendency to pull back. . . . If a parent is a real creep, I'm not going to remember that the kid is a different person.

Another mother agreed: "If I come across as a real bitch, then that could prejudice some people against my kid." The fear that their actions might jeopardize future opportunities to obtain any help thus exaggerated the insecurity and self-doubt associated with the stage of disenchantment.

Fear of repercussions was sufficient to prevent some of these patients and families from acting out their frustration. As one patient explained, "You're not supposed to make waves. And also, you don't know if . . . in some way this is going to jeopardize your care." For those unable to express frustration openly, disenchantment was a time of hopelessness and despair. One woman explained, "I was so mad at my MD, you know, I was so mad I was going to bawl him out. But what's the use of that because I have to go to him?" At times like these, people described themselves as being overwhelmed with guilt and self-doubt.

In the stage of disenchantment, some chronically ill individuals and families tried to find solace in rationalizing their experiences as "bad luck" or by attempting to take personal responsibility for what had happened to them. One woman's soul-searching illustrates such efforts.

> I'm beginning to think it's just me. I've done it with four of them [doctors].
> But that's not the way my relationships are normally with other people. I'm
> not that kind of person that usually goes around being an adversary, or
> combative-type person.

Another man expressed similar introspection: "I started to question myself, 'What is wrong with me?' " According to the accounts, many of these patients and families believed that any explanation of what was happening to them would be preferable to the dreadful possibility that their previous assumptions about health care professionals might have been unfounded.

The emotional disruption that characterized disenchantment was later interpreted by patients and families as a logical outcome of their early naiveté and ignorance. They later understood their actions and responses during this stage in terms of being unable to either make sense of or control any meaningful aspect of their situation. For example, one man recalled his overwhelming sense of being out of control. "It's really tough when you can see no way out. You can just see this cloud over your head—just sort of for the rest of your life, that there's no help, there's nothing."

The feelings associated with disenchantment were sufficiently unpleasant that they made it difficult for these people to remain in this stage for any extended period of time. As one woman observed, "Desperation is the right word." Their level of distress, in combination with the realization that ongoing health care was essential, provided an incentive to do something to resolve the adversarial relationships. As one patient's thoughts illustrate, the intense frustration in disenchantment was especially difficult in combination with a profound and desperate sense of dependence: "How can I be so critical of the whole medical profession when I have to rely on them? My whole being needs them!"

Thus, disenchantment was a stage in the evolution of health care relationships emerging out of shattered naive and lofty ideals of what an ongoing health care relationship would consist of. Having placed absolute faith in professional health care providers, the chronically ill and their families were inevitably disillusioned by the limitations and failures of the health care professionals in whom they had placed their trust.

Guarded Alliance

The transition into the third stage, guarded alliance, was generally triggered by a series of insights about the situation in which these patients and families found themselves. One such insight was that health care professionals are part of a larger health care system with its own inherent set of values and assumptions.

> I mean, just hearing about the things like useless surgeries, and not taking a preventative approach, and all that . . . I guess, I'm in double minds. One is that there's an incredible amount of knowledge and resources out there. I mean, there's just an endless amount of skills that are out there. And I think what I am negative about is that I don't think it's able to be utilized very effectively by a large number of people, and that's the hardest part. I mean, you either have to be really assertive, and really articulate, or very lucky!

Thus, they began to shift their analysis away from a focus on the qualities of an individual professional and toward an understanding of that professional's part in a larger system.

A related insight was that they were capable of making choices about their health care experience without jeopardizing health care relationships more than they had done so already. As one patient explained, "You have to do all the mental head trips about, you know, who you are and what you have a right to do, like your own advocacy kind of thing. And so it's not spontaneous and easy. You just have to work at it." As another patient observed, "I accepted the fact that any change that's going to be made is mostly made by us."

In recognizing the constraints of the traditional health care system, these patients and families freed themselves to consider that there were alternatives to unconditional and passive adherence. Thus, their profound confusion was replaced by new understanding of how their own experience might fit into the larger picture of health care delivery; further, their self-doubt was transformed into a suspicion that they might actually have some important competencies that could be applied to their health problem. As one informant commented, "That maybe would have been the pivotal point of attitude change for me, that hey, I'm doing something for myself!" By locating their individual experience within the context of the larger picture, these people were able to make order out of chaos and meaning out of their experience with disenchantment.

In guarded alliance, a variety of ways were employed by patients and families to make sense of and manage their health care relationships. They used numerous creative and effective mechanisms toward reconstructing the shattered trust between them and their health care professionals. Characteristic of guarded alliance was a distinct shift in attitudes about their own responsibility for health care relationships. Through analysis of their own experiences with health care providers, focusing this time not on their own inadequacies but on the limitations of the professionals, they learned of the importance of such responsibility. As one informant noted:

> I think I had to get over that psychological barrier of they're in charge of my physical well-being—when I go to see them I'm putting myself into their hands. I had to have a behavioral change from that to the point where I was saying, "Hey, I'm in charge of it."

Because chronic illness management was a matter of living with it as much as treating it, these patients and families eventually recognized that they had, in fact, become the experts.

> They weren't in my life. I mean, they would go home after work, and everything was fine. They didn't have problems like I had. I mean, they knew of it, they saw it all the time, but that still didn't make them experts at it.

The patients and families living with chronic illness came to recognize not only that responsibility for health care was theirs by default, but also that they did have genuine capabilities with which to address this responsibility. These capabilities were seen as something quite distinct from the expert knowledge and authority of the health care professional. As one patient explained, "It was more a sense of growing power within me to make my own decisions that evolved out of the frustration." Thus, they could accept responsibility without denying the expertise of the professionals in certain arenas. As one woman remarked, "The medical profession was really helpful in dealing with the acute phases of it. But there was nothing, really, that helped me in dealing with the long-term problems."

The second major insight associated with the stage of guarded alliance was the realization by patients and families that health care professionals were seriously limited in their ability to provide meaningful services to the chronically ill. At this stage, they began to understand that their disappointments with health care professionals were far from unique. By generalizing their interpretations beyond their own experience, these patients and families developed a broader understanding about how health care operated.

The chronically ill individuals and families offered various explanations for these limitations. Some blamed the system's inadequacies on the inflated expectations of patients. As one commented, "Like, I think people place doctors on little pedestals, and they're way up there, and they forget that they're human." Others believed that professional education was a contributing problem. "They're all learning, most of them. Like you might get somebody to sew your kid up that doesn't know how to sew too good or something." In addition, many informants began to understand that the behavior of health care professionals was motivated by an understandable anxiety about the legal implications of their actions. As one man commented, "If you put your foot down, I'm sure they'll do it [send you to a specialist], mainly because of all sorts of liability, you know. They can't bamboozle you anymore. People are getting too sophisticated." Another explained, "I think they're preserving themselves . . . they really see themselves as protecting themselves rather than being there for the patient."

On the basis of these key insights, patients and families in guarded alliance reconstructed some form of trust within the context of a health care relationship. Because they had recognized the system's limitations and considered the patient's responsibility, these people were now able to rebuild a form of trust founded upon a different set of expectations and a renewed sense of confidence. In contrast to the less conscious cognitive shifts that had taken place in naive trust and in disenchantment, the reconstruction of trust in guarded alliance was the product of a deliberate decision to adopt a new attitude toward health care relationships. This reconstructed trust permitted people to continue seeking help without abandoning the insights they had gained from their experiences in the previous stages. As one man explained:

> If I made my judgments on the basis of the negative experiences I've had with the health care system, and condemned all the individuals in it . . . first of all, I wouldn't still be going to them, second of all, I probably would've cut myself off from some things that have helped me. . . . I'm glad that I have been sensitized to some of the weaknesses, so that it's not just that slavish adherence to it.

Reconstructed trust differed from naive trust in that it was highly selective, depending on the specific criteria which each patient and family member considered important. One woman, for example, explained that she sought professionals who could tolerate criticism of the system. Others had not been sufficiently fortunate to find such exceptional professionals, but expressed the belief that such individuals might exist. As one woman commented, "I think they're in the minority, but I know there are some out there." Trust in an individual rather than in a system reflected many patients' and families' increasing confidence in their own judgment about what was meaningful in health care relationships.

Even as they expressed a sincere trust for a specific health care provider, the informants also acknowledged that there were definite limitations to that trust. For example, informants now recognized that health care providers had human failings. As one woman said, "Like, now I trust [Dr. B.] and what he says. But I still think that he's a human being, and he could make errors." These patients and families also recognized specific limitations in the service they could expect from their professional health care providers, as one woman's comments illustrate: "I trust [my doctors] on the level we're at. If there's another big change in the illness again, I don't know if I'd be that same way."

By reconstructing a new form of trust, patients and families were able to regain optimism and comfort in their health care relationships. Their ability to analyze their trust revealed the insights inherent in guarded alliance. As one patient explained, "I used to feel really strong that the system was abusive, and uncaring, and sort of controlling of my life,

but I don't feel so much that way now. I guess I've come through that."
Thus, the stage of guarded alliance represented a resolution to the
frustration and confusion of disenchantment by permitting a more
informed and conditional trust in health professionals.

VARIATIONS IN RECONSTRUCTED TRUST

Once they had achieved guarded alliance, the chronically ill individuals
and family members in this study were certainly not immune to anger or
despair. However, their new understanding prevented them from experiencing the intense confusion that characterized disenchantment. They now
had a framework for making sense of what was happening in their health
care relationships and for taking action to make such relationships function
more effectively. As these men and women explained their health care
relationships in this stage, four distinct patterns became evident: hero
worship, resignation, consumerism, and team playing (Thorne & Robinson, 1989). Although each pattern represented an alliance of some sort,
guarded by a generalized or specific awareness of limitations, there were
obvious differences in the types of health care relationships they permitted.
In this discussion, the characteristics of each of the four patterns will be
described in some detail.

At first, the four relationship types appeared as personality traits or
coping styles peculiar to each patient or family; later, the discovery that
most people actually engaged in various types of relationships over
time, or in multiple relationships of different types concurrently, challenged this initial assumption. Further, ongoing data analysis revealed
that there was no absolute hierarchy of preferred relationship types.
While many patients and families claimed a preference for certain kinds
of relationships, they also explained the advantages of other types at
different points in their ongoing illness experience. Thus, the four
variations seem to reflect more or less strategic options for managing
the inherent problems of health care relationships in chronic illness.

Hero Worship

In relationships characterized by hero worship, the chronically ill
patients and families identified one individual health care professional
who was different from all others and therefore worthy of absolute trust.
Thus, hero worship allowed for insights about the limitations of health

care professionals in general while it simultaneously permitted people to regain the comfort and security of a strong trust. In order for a professional to be granted hero status, he or she had to be perceived as different from other professionals. This special status could be conferred on the basis of special clinical expertise, as one man explained:

> I wouldn't trust anybody else, but I trust [my doctor]. You know, he knows what he's talking about. He just does knee joints. And, you know, I'm a carpenter, and if I just specialize in putting windows in a house, I'm going to get pretty good at putting windows in a house, right? So if he's opened up enough knees that he's seen different knees and you know what they're like.

Alternatively, the professional's special status could derive from his or her reputation. As one woman remarked, "I trust him very much, because he's definitely a top man in his field." However, in many cases, what informants found special about their hero was not his or her clinical expertise per se; rather, it was some more personal quality that caused the professional to depart from the norm in the patient or family's perspective. Such attributes as effective listening, a cheerful attitude, remembering names, and taking the time to chat were frequently mentioned as evidence of the special qualities of a particular hero. As one man explained, "When he's talking to you, he's there maybe for 5 minutes, but it seems like 15. Whereas other doctors, they're there for 5 minutes, and it seems like 2."

While clinical competencies and communication skills were popular explanations for a hero's special nature, there were many instances in which the differences articulated were less clearly related to clinical practice. For example, one professional was considered special because he came from the prairies; another, because his father had been a well-known socialist. One hero was described as different by virtue of being an ex-hippie; another, because he refused to wear a lab coat in the office. Some heroes played at a prestigious golf course or had excellent collegial connections. Others lived a life-style that the patient could identify with, as one woman's explanation illustrates:

> I think he has a better understanding of what his patients go through because he seems a very normal kind of person. He lives in this community, his son plays soccer, and I see him at soccer games and baseball games. And he's involved with Scouts, and his wife and I worked together with Guides and Brownies. And I see them as very close to how his patients live.

Thus, those professionals identified as heroes were distinguished from their colleagues by some criterion of personal significance to the chronically ill patients and their families.

Hero worship produced a precarious dependence on one individual health care professional. One woman, for example, described her reaction to the news that her hero was leaving practice. She said, "I just really panicked almost, 'cause it was just like my life support system, you know. What am I going to do?" Thus the comfort of having a hero was qualified somewhat by the anxiety of being overly dependent on one rather special health care professional.

In hero worship relationships, patients and families described themselves as putting the health care professional on a pedestal. Having located their hero, they placed themselves in his or her hands and accepted whatever decisions were made on their behalf. In some instances, this form of reconstructed trust was so wholehearted that it resembled naive trust. On further exploration, however, it was always distinguishable by the presence of general dissatisfactions about the health care system from which the hero was exempt. Thus, it represented a strategic means by which these ill individuals and families could enjoy the reassurance of being able to trust, without ignoring the frustrating realities associated with health care in general.

Resignation

A second and markedly different type of relationship was termed "resignation" because of its characteristic submissiveness, negativity, and hopelessness. In this pattern, the patients and families engaged in health care relationships but felt little optimism about what they could offer. As one patient explained, "There's nobody there to help me. I really believe that now." Their frustrations with health care produced an atmosphere of depression and despair. Although this state seemed somewhat like a chronic form of disenchantment, it was distinguishable by virtue of the fact that patients and families in these relationships understood what was happening and why.

Such insights, however, offered little comfort. In resignation, the problems in health care seemed too large for the chronically ill to tackle alone, and so they felt compelled to continue on in health care relationships in which they had little faith, as one woman's comments illustrate:

> Right now it's not sufficiently bad. Like she's not medically mismanaging me. She's just being . . . as far as I'm concerned, she's acting like a

doctor. . . . But it seems to me that all of life is a trade-off. And probably if I found somebody that I really liked, they'd have such a horrendously big practice that I would not get access or something.

In some cases, informants withdrew from health care completely for a period of time. As one woman angrily remarked, "I don't need anybody's help now, because they haven't given it to me in the last 15 years. Why in the hell would they start now?" Interestingly, this woman had recently lost a hero worshipping health care relationship and, during the course of the study, was able to find a second hero in which to place her trust.

While declarations of complete withdrawal were common, the accounts suggested that most people did not abstain from health care relationships for long. Instead, they usually went through the motions without any real expectations of service.

> After a while, some people give up and they say, "Well, I don't care." They make an appointment with the doctor. They show up there. As a matter of fact, I did that. And you try to cheat the doctor as much as you can, because you don't want anything to do with the doctor, but you go there, right?

Although such resigned health care relationships were quite unsatisfying, they did serve the purpose of representing a form of "insurance" against the event of health care situations in which an alliance with a professional was required. As one man explained:

> I go in for regular blood tests. I check in periodically and let them know how things are going. It's just so they're updated on everything, so if anything really goes bad, well, they saw me a couple of months ago and they know how it's going. I don't expect a lot out of them.

And one woman noted:

> One of the reasons I keep having a doctor and keep my medical up to date is because I know that eventually my mother will die and I know that all kinds of complications will happen if she doesn't have a physician to come and sign the death certificate.

Thus, patients and families in relationships characterized by resignation continued their involvement with professionals, but for reasons unique to their own situation. As one patient explained, "I would say that I just wrote the system off and refused to participate, but I'm still leery enough to keep my medical [insurance] up to date, just in case."

Beyond staying involved with professionals, resignation included a pervasive sense of powerlessness as to their own ability to effect changes in their unfortunate situation. One woman's comments illustrate such a feeling of futility. "You get to thinking, 'Well, what's the use?' You know what he's going to say, so what can you do? Change doctors again? *(laugh)* I'm running out of doctors!" Often, the patients and families suspected that the health care professional was equally powerless and frustrated with the situation.

> I would think it frustrated them more than it did me. I always thought, "Poor Dr. M." One reason I don't go in there very often. He's a very nice man, but I feel how frustrating for him—a physician—being able to do nothing.

While most resigned relationships indicated times of powerlessness and despair among the chronically ill and their families, there were instances in which they reflected an acceptable and sometimes even constructive strategic response. For example, several people described such relationships as a "time out" from the intense involvement required to maintain other types of health care relationships. Because struggling with health care relationships could be a constant reminder that they were ill, some patients and families used resignation as a break from focusing intensively on their chronic illness. Thus, even this most depressing and unpleasant relationship type sometimes represented a strategic alternative with regard to reconstructing trust in guarded alliance.

Consumerism

In contrast to the passivity of resignation, consumerism represented a relationship characterized by a more active service orientation on the part of the ill individuals and families. Instead of focusing on the relationship per se, consumers concentrated on the service they needed and developed strategies to work with the health care professional in order to increase their likelihood of obtaining those services. As one man stated, "I treat the medical profession as a service in one respect. I mean, if you look at it in a very clinical way—excuse that expression—then it is a service." Another patient articulated a similarly functional perspective. "I just treat them the same way as if you ran out of gas in your car and you saw a Safeway store. Safeway store's no good if you need gas!"

In this type of relationship, the patients and families no longer expected health care professionals to attend to the real needs of their clients. As one woman commented, "They're there for one specific role and that's it. And I'm sure they forget your face, although they may remember your incision." However, they had learned that needed services could only be obtained through apparent cooperation with a professional health care provider, as one woman noted: "You see, I can't prescribe my own medication. I am dependent on her to get that. So I have to do what she says. I have to follow her instruction if I'm going to fill my needs." Another consumer summarized his attitude toward health care professionals: "Oh, they're a necessary evil, aren't they!" Thus, consumerism represented a conscious strategy to convince health care professionals to provide what services were available. As one man theorized, "I guess you become a professional doctor visitor."

The consumer relationship allowed chronically ill individuals and their families to turn their frustration with health care professionals into a source of insight into professional attitudes, which they then used to manipulate the health care professionals. As one patient explained, "You learn to ask questions, and when to and when not to, and stuff like that." Another commented, "I go into every situation defensive, expecting the worst, and then I take it from there." Still another individual admitted:

> There's a certain sense that if you hype it up about the critical nature of it, that you're going to command a greater response. And that's a really nasty dynamic happening. . . . And I have to admit that, at times, I have hyped up the condition that I have in order to get adequate treatment.

Another patient claimed to have manufactured a rash as a means of obtaining a sufficient supply of prescribed medication to enjoy a trouble-free holiday.

> You see, you can play the system. You might put that in there [the research report]. Hey, I'm not doing anything wrong. It's not a lie. I really do break out in this rash once in a while, and, who knows, I'm probably allergic to the kids, right? I don't know. And I really do have the Crohn's. It's been diagnosed by an internist. I'm not making this up. Just the fact that they all come together at the same time, and that I happen to have a plane ticket to go somewhere—hey!

Similarly, another patient reported manipulating test results to avoid a treatment plan with which she was not comfortable.

He suggested that I would probably be put on Prednisone because these other forms of medications were not controlling it in the way that he wanted it to be controlled. So I, in fact, cheated on one of my lung function tests. And I told a lie.

These manipulative and defensive strategies were clearly derived from the perceptions of these patients and families about what was necessary in order to obtain the health care they required. However, because obtaining service was foremost in the minds of these consumers, they were most anxious that health professionals not discover their duplicity. Therefore, they claimed to behave as if they trusted the professionals while maintaining as much control as they could of all health care decisions.

While the consumer relationship often included ongoing frustration and anger on the part of the patient and family, it differed from resignation in that they recognized and acted on a perception that they had power within the system. For example, many patients and family members recognized that they could establish their own standards as to what they would accept from health care professionals. As one man explained,

In terms of personal health care, it's, you know, buyer beware, and a consumer's marketplace. And if I'm willing to sit around and be satisfied with second-rate stuff, then that's my problem. And it will not be a problem, there's no doubt in my mind.

These men and women also understood that they had the option not to be intimidated by their interactions with health care professionals. As one patient remarked, "I think the doctor is a person no better than I am, but informed and knowledgeable in areas that I'm not and I need. But I'm not scared to say anything to them, whether it be nice or not nice."

In order to be effective in a consumer relationship, informants required considerable knowledge about their illness and its treatment. Many relied upon outside sources of information, such as support groups, institutes, and other professionals, to develop such knowledge. Several taught themselves how to get access to and evaluate the professional literature housed in the local university's biomedical library. Others kept up on recent research developments through careful monitoring of magazine, newspaper, and television reports. In addition, many informed themselves about alternative treatment modalities and philosophies. These patients and families described extensive knowledge as requisite to their success in consumer relationships, as one woman's explanation illustrates:

I've been doing lots of personal experimenting around this stuff, and I feel like I'm getting a handle on it. And it gives me a sense of more control. I need these people. I need these specialists. I need to pick their brains. But I don't believe there's anybody out there, and I don't care what their degree is, knows my metabolism or the things that are going to trigger it as well as I'm going to get to know it if I start making the time to tune in.

Consumerism was therefore a comfortable relationship type for many patients and families. Because they had to rely on their own skill and ingenuity to acquire necessary services, these people developed confidence in their ability to make decisions and to manage their own health care. As one woman stated, "I've detached myself from that nonsense. And I don't want to be back in their hands, because you lose your self-control in that sense." To be sure, some consumers remained regretful that they could not trust a health care professional. They claimed that considerable energy was required for this constant vigilance and control over decisions. Further, many of the patients and family members missed the sense of security that comes from knowing that they could really trust someone. As one man scornfully remarked, "They're just note takers and monitorists."

Thus, consumerism afforded chronically ill individuals and their families considerable control over the management of their health care and, consequently, over the quality of their chronic illness experience. In turn, however, it required that they accept an enormous responsibility without the security of trusting in professional health care support.

Team Playing

The final type of guarded alliance reflected a reciprocal and negotiative relationship between those living with chronic illness and their professional health care providers. As in hero worship, the team players aligned themselves with individual health care professionals whom they considered different from the norm. As in consumerism, they were able to develop and apply their own knowledge in health care decision making. Thus, for many, team playing represented a kind of ideal.

In order for team playing to be successful, the limitations of mainstream health care had to be acknowledged and accepted by both the patients and the professionals, as one man explained:

Now I've got a doctor that helps me understand that I have to make a contribution to my own well-being, that listens first to my problems and personalizes it, that I can have a little fun with, and still get medical help. And yet I'm realistic enough to know that he is still operating within the traditional medical system, and there is only so many things he can do for me. That's why it is a good relationship that I have with him right now, because it's positive, and its limitations are clear.

This stance required that patients and families accept personal responsibility for many aspects of their health care. Creating and nourishing team playing relationships also required considerable effort on their part, as one man explained:

I've sort of insisted on it being a sort of copartnership kind of thing, at the same time as not trying to—I mean, you know, stroking their professional ego whenever necessary. And that's the negative way of saying it, but I mean allowing the respect of their area of expertise but still, you know, we're in this together.

In addition, team playing required that the professionals be comfortable admitting to the limits of medical science and respecting the potential contribution of alternative or nontraditional approaches to illness care. Since, as could be predicted, professionals capable of such admissions were rare, genuine team playing relationships were not considered easy to find. Team playing also required that the distinct contributions of patients and professionals be recognized and valued by both parties. As one woman explained, "You're both involved in this. They from their expertise and you from your personal experience." Another woman described her delight at finding a professional capable of such attitudes: "Here is a human being with all these degrees, and he's asking me! You see, he's fairly young, he's only about 38 years old. He's not set in his ways like a lot of these old, you know, three-piece-suiters!"

Thus, team playing represented a satisfying reciprocal relationship between health care recipients and professionals. As one woman commented, "I feel I have a right to reciprocate. . . . I feel it sort of puts us on the same level." They described such relationships as collaborative and directed toward mutually agreeable goals. One woman quoted her doctor as saying, "We're investigators, you and I, to really find out what we can work with and what fits together." Another explained:

I call that collaboration, because it's a change in my realization of my own role as part of this team. Whereas before, I didn't see myself as being part of that team. I saw myself as going to the team for help for [my daughter]. And now I see myself as an integral part.

Reciprocity in the team playing relationship required mutual trust. Patients and their families had to be willing to trust a health care professional, and health care professionals had to trust their clients as competent people. As one patient explained it, "Trust me, and I will trust you."

For many of the patients and families in this study, finding a suitable health care professional could be the most frustrating aspect of team playing relationships. One woman outlined the strategy that she had developed to assess a professional's team playing capacity.

I'm going to tell him the very first day that I have a bad reputation with rheumatologists, and that I like to be involved in the process, and that I hope he will involve me. I don't want to dictate. I haven't got his education. But I just want to be part of it.

Another patient had devised a similar plan.

I thought I'd go up and at least have a chat with him, and see what he's like. Might as well go to him for something minor, and see if I like the fellow or not. But I went in there with the attitude that I'm not going to sit here and go yes sir, yes sir. I went in with the attitude that here's the situation, have you got any suggestions as to what we can do about this? And my attitude was, what are we going to do together? Don't just tell me what to do.

Aside from the difficulty in finding a suitable professional with whom to form a team, these patients and families noted one additional drawback to such relationships. From their perspective, the intensity of effort to stay sufficiently well-informed for full participation in decision making could be exhausting and draining. Thus, while successful team playing relationships were usually productive and comfortable for patients and their families, they were not always possible and, in some cases, not always ideal.

Thus, guarded alliance, a stage that represents the resolution of inevitable conflictual experiences in health care relationships, can be conceptualized as including four distinct types of relationships between ongoing health care recipients and their professional health care providers. As has been evident in the accounts of these patients and families, each relationship type demands certain conditions. Further, each has its own unique strengths and limitations.

DISCUSSION

The accounts of the chronically ill individuals and family members in this study illustrate the importance of health care relationships in shaping the chronic illness experience. They depict such relationships as evolving through three stages toward a state in which some measure of trust can be constructed on the basis of new insights about two central issues: the limitations of the health care system, and the responsibilities that befall the chronically ill and their families.

According to the men and women involved in this process, conflict between prior romantic expectations and the realities of health care relationships is inevitable in chronic illness. The scholarly literature provides considerable evidence that this phenomenon is widespread. For example, Duff, a student of decision making in health care, has claimed that such ongoing health care relationships are characterized by "evasions, half-truths, and lies" (1988, p. 211).

> What counts as a "right and good healing action" is easy to see when a sickness can be cured, or when no sickness exists and the patient simply requires reassurance that this is so. But, when sickness is more or less chronic, we cannot understand a right and good healing action without understanding what the sickness is doing to the person's self-respect, to his life plan, and to the narrative account of his life. (Brody, 1987, p. 192)

However, Barnard reports that, "For most of medicine's modern history, physicians have distrusted patients' views of their own experience" (1988, p. 90).

Mizrahi (1986) offers an explanation, rooted in the socialization process of medical education, for the behavior of physicians. According to his research, the superordinate objective of the medical resident can be summarized with the phrase "getting rid of patients." Because medical education teaches the students to value quick technical solutions, health care relationships are often relegated to the status of "sociological bullshit" (p. 118). As such, they are seen to interfere with the "real" work of medicine. Mechanic (1979b) notes that the increased bureaucratization of health care over recent decades has also diluted the professional's sense of personal responsibility for health care relationships. Further, Pritchard (1983) suggests that the professional assumption equating increased approachability with loss of power may have factored in maintaining distance within health care relationships.

As has been noted by others, creating and maintaining satisfactory health care relationships is considered a major adaptive task for those confronting chronic illness (Ben-Sira, 1984; Moos & Tsu, 1977). The literature also indicates that negotiative and collaborative health care relationship models are especially valued by chronically ill individuals and their families (Kleinman et al., 1978; MacElveen-Hoehn, 1983). While the informants in this study often preferred such relationship forms, their accounts made it clear that they were often unavailable because of certain attitudes and values on the part of professionals. As has been pointed out by others, such an empathetic and cooperative model is "essentially foreign to medicine" (Szasz & Hollender, 1980, p. 322). Further, the informants indicated that there were circumstances or occasions in which the work involved in sustaining such relationships could be too taxing for the patient and family. These informants challenged the notion of a fixed ideal in health care relationships, suggesting instead a variety of strengths and limitations to several relationship models.

The accounts create a rich description of the importance of health care relationships in chronic illness. They illustrate some of the complexities of such relationships and highlight some of the predictable patterns and variations within them. Further, they point to serious problems within health care that render such relationships conflictual and unsatisfying.

Trust and Confidence

The previous chapter presented the argument that health care relationships in chronic illness evolve through three predictable stages before taking on one of four discrete patterns. By considering the experience of the chronically ill from their perspective, it generated a description of the importance of health care relationships within the chronic illness experience. Further, it brought forth the message that such relationships could be highly problematic to patients and their families. In this chapter, two central themes in such relationships will be examined in further detail. This examination will permit analysis of the best and the worst of ongoing health care relationships, preparing a foundation for subsequent discussion of pieces which will contribute to the larger puzzle of chronic illness experience.

The types of relationships that have been observed between chronically ill people and their professional health care providers reflect variations with regard to two dimensions of such relationships: the degree to which trust in a professional is possible, and the degree to which confidence in the patient's and family's own competence can be attained. By plotting these dimensions on intersecting axes, their utility in accounting for the variance between the four guarded alliance relationship configurations can be illustrated.

While the discussion in the previous chapter hinted at some of the ways in which the relationship types differed from one another, this will focus analysis on the dimensions that appeared to explain these distinctions. In so doing, it will present the interpretations of patients and families about the conditions under which their trust in an individual professional health care provider is made possible and desirable, as well as the circumstances under which their confidence in their own judgment about health care management issues is made viable.

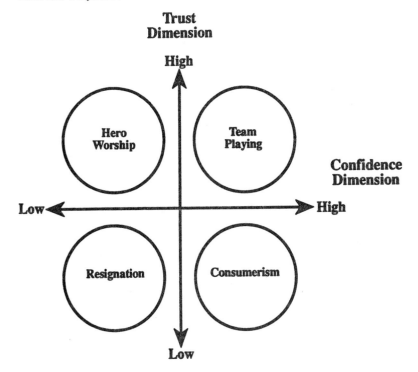

Figure 6.1. Guarded Alliance Model

SOURCE: Adapted from Thorne, S. E., & Robinson, C. A. (1989). Guarded alliance: Health care relationships in chronic illness. *Image: The Journal of Nursing Scholarship, 21,* 153-157. Reprinted with permission.

TRUSTWORTHY PROFESSIONALS

Team playing and hero worship relationships required that the patient and family find a professional health care provider worthy of their trust. Further, they demanded a willingness to trust a professional to make appropriate decisions on their behalf. Since naive trust had been shattered, this new trust represented a conscious determination to try again in a more informed way. For some people, the risks of trusting were too great, leaving a consumer relationship as the preferred option. For others, the appeal of a trusting relationship was powerful, and considerable attention was focused on creating one. The accounts of how such relationships were discovered, created, and sustained reveal the astute analyses of the informants about themselves, the professionals, and the conditions under which they interact.

The Nature of Trustworthiness

The accounts revealed that health care professional trustworthiness was comprised of a combination of competence and communication skills. While few patients and families considered themselves adequately informed to judge competence according to the usual standards associated with formal licensing or membership in a professional association, many had strong convictions about the issue of competence. Their evaluations of competence reflected recognition of technical skill, clinical reasoning, and other elements of expert practice. Further, as earlier chapters have illustrated, a surprisingly large number of informants believed that they had seen evidence of incompetence at some point in their chronic illness careers. For example, one woman pointed to overprescription as an example of incompetence. She said, "Every time I went to see my doctor he would prescribe a pill. . . . Some doctors prescribe so many. One man I know, he told me he takes 16 pills a day! That's crazy! And he's always sick."

The second ingredient for trust involved the personality and communication skills of the individual health care professional. From the perspective of these patients and families, certain qualities were consistent with trustworthy behavior on the part of these professionals. Examination of the accounts concerning these qualities illustrates the way in which informants evaluated communication for evidence of trustworthiness.

Among the most important communication skills described by these informants was active listening. As one recalled, "The nurses were great. . . . They'd come in and talk to you if you wanted to talk. If you wanted to cry, they'd sit and listen to you." Another explained:

> It's not that I just need to sit there and rap with somebody about my problems. I want to be heard. I want somebody who will listen to me. I want somebody who is sensitive to the fact that I have a problem.

Further, they were impressed by professionals who could explain things to them in a respectful yet understandable manner, as one woman noted:

> When you're going into something like this, you expect them to talk in complete medical terms. She took it down to a level where everybody could understand it . . . she spoke in such a manner that everybody understood.

The patients and families favored those health care professionals who understood the importance of talking about and understanding what was happening to them. Such interaction was appreciated as a source of both information and comfort. Without this type of interaction, competence was insufficient for trust, as one informant's characterization of her physician illustrates:

> He reminds me of the type or person that's—how shall I say this—well, as a child, he would probably be the brain in his class and socially he wouldn't get along with people. You can talk to him, but it was always businesslike.

Thus, from their perspective, competence was worthwhile only if the professional had the time or inclination to apply it to their cases.

Willingness to learn was also a highly valued professional attribute, according to these patients and families. One mother of a child with PKU remembered such willingness on the part of a new physician. "He said to her that he was glad to have her for a patient, because he had never had one that was PKU, and therefore he would be able to learn from her." Especially among older patients, an important quality within health care relationships was willingness to take time. One woman commented, "Now I see Dr. H., and I think he's wonderful. You go in, and he's not in any hurry. He'll talk to you." In contrast, most patients found professionals rather impatient. "He's a man that moves quickly, talks quickly, thinks quickly, and everything happens quickly."

The patients and families also valued professionals with a sense of perspective on what living with a chronic illness might be like. One mother offered the following anecdote to illustrate such perspective from her physician:

> I said to my family doctor at one point, "I'm going to kill her. I'm going to take this kid, and I'm going to smash her head into a wall, and there's going to be nothing left of her." And I'll never forget it, because he sat in the office and he laughed at me, and he said, "No, you won't, because you know you want to, and therefore you won't do it." . . . And sometimes I think that's more important than all the medical garbage they can give you. You know, anybody can give you medical statistics . . . but you need somebody there who's going to pick up on you as a person.

Another patient recalled a similar sense of perspective that allowed his doctor to empathize effectively. "I'll go in and he'll say, 'You know, this is really a shitty disease to have, isn't it?' And I just know he knows that's how I'm feeling."

Being willing to forgo formalities was described by many patients and families as critical to trusting health care relationships. For many people, being on a first name basis symbolized disinterest in perpetuating the traditional power imbalance in health care relationships. As one patient commented, "Like I feel I could call him by his first name. He's not on the pedestal; he's lounging around on the couch with me." Similarly, most people appreciated health care professionals who were willing to reveal something of their own individual identity. For many patients and families, key details of personal information helped them to connect with the human qualities of the health care professional. For example, one man was impressed by his doctor's political leanings and previous civic activities. And one mother found it comforting to know that her doctor also had teenage children. "He can really understand that because he's got teenagers too . . . and they're going through the same sort of a thing." From their perspective, such personal information helped to reduce the artificial social separations between patient and professional.

Among the most valued qualities in positive health care relationships was a health care professional's respect for the patient as a unique individual. One man's account illustrates such respect:

> And the first time I went in to him, I told him, "Now look, if I ever get into a life-threatening position—heart, or whatever—and I find out that you ever put any lifesaving devices on me," I said, "When I do go, my spirit'll come back and haunt you the rest of your life." He looked at me, he said, "You put that in writing." I said, "For certain." He brought in one of his office staff, and typed it out, and that's what heads my medical file . . . so that any doctor knows what my feeling is on the subject.

Another patient explained that such respect required that they be treated "like a person" and not "like a disease." According to these patients and families, respect was not so much a matter of politeness as it was a reflection of genuine appreciation of the client as a competent person. As one remarked, "Now that sort of thing I appreciate from a doctor. He doesn't hesitate to bawl the living daylights out of me every time he sees me about smoking." And another explained, "She doesn't treat me like your standard sickie." Being believed by the professional was integral to such respect. As one woman noted, "There are some doctors who feel—that are actually concerned about you. And they take your word for it. They don't consider you a neurotic fool."

In addition to such qualities, accessibility was an important component of trustworthiness for informants. As one young mother explained, she "wouldn't have survived" without the easy access to a wonderful dietitian during the first year of her child's chronic illness. "She was a crutch, I guess, in a way, but it was a crutch that I needed." While easy access to professionals was infrequent, people often described situations in which they believed that certain professionals had given them access beyond what would be necessary to demonstrate concern for their patients. Because they were rare, such acts were always reported with awe and with admiration.

Thus, these informants explained qualities that they considered integral to trustworthiness in health care relationships. Their accounts illustrated examples of excellence in communication, respect, concern, and humility on the part of some professionals. They emphasized the human qualities within health care relationships as the foundation for a reconstructed trust. Further, they suggest that chronically ill patients and families have a consistent vision of what excellence entails in this regard.

Strategic Trust-Building

While the patients and families shared a vision of what trust in health care relationships entailed, they also found that it was rather difficult to achieve. Therefore, they generated strategies with which to find a trustworthy professional or create a trusting relationship. For some, this involved finding a professional with the appropriate raw materials; for others, it meant devising means by which to maximize the trustworthy behaviors in the professional they already had.

When efforts to build trust in existing health care relationships were unsuccessful or undesirable, many patients and families advocated "doctor shopping" as a critical strategy. Although they recognized that changing doctors was generally frowned upon by health care professionals, many people came to believe that it was necessary. As one patient remarked, "If I see somebody who isn't interested in my input, or my questions or anything, then I just don't continue with them, you know. I just fire them and find somebody else!" The process of shopping for a health professional required that patients and families have a clear idea of what they required and sufficient confidence to act on their own behalf, despite the disapproval of others. "Well, you sort of have to think of yourself sometimes first. Who cares if their feelings are hurt? I'm willing to give them a couple of chances, but it's my life!"

However competent and caring a health care professional might be, the lessons of disenchantment had led most patients and families to believe that professional knowledge and skill were unevenly applied, favoring those patients in whom the professional took special interest. For this reason, many people explained that it was useful to devise ways of creating the kind of interaction that would appeal to the professional. For example, one woman talked of giving her health care professionals positive feedback to show appreciation and to encourage continued interest. "I just write them all cards. . . . If they're nice I write them and say, you know, 'It's really good to know you're out there, and I appreciate your knowledge.' " Others described gift-giving as a means of sustaining the professional's interest in their case. Thus, one important strategy for building trust was to create the type of interaction that the professional would remember and value.

Another strategy for building trust included empathizing with the role and conditions of the health care professional. Overwork and understaffing were among those conditions reported as frustrating the efforts of the professionals. As one patient observed, "I know that they're understaffed and there aren't enough nurses and they don't have enough time either." Many patients and families also empathized with the difficulties inherent in working with sick people.

> I figure when you keep seeing people who are sick all the time and, you know, especially someone who may be really at the end of their life—like medical people have to put up fences, too, right? I mean they can't just get involved with every single person or they just couldn't do the job.

At the same time as they expressed considerable sympathy for those who worked in health care, many of these patients and families doubted whether these conditions were sufficient to explain the behavior of some professionals. As one woman pointedly asked, "Does the professional pride wear out after a while, or does it get tired?" Understanding of the role and conditions of health care permitted patients and families to develop strategies whereby they could demonstrate respect and concern for the professional. Further, it also provided them with a basis for identifying when intervention within the relationship could be appropriate. As one man explained:

> A couple of times, I thought he was maybe just beginning to lose a little bit of credibility in me as a real credible patient, you know. Not in a big

way, but at one point I thought that maybe he was just losing a bit. He wasn't quite as behind me. I wrote a 10-page letter detailing my thoughts about the whole thing. Every kind of point that I could think of. After that, he couldn't do enough for me.

Thus, the patients and families used their understanding of the conditions under which health care professionals practiced to generate a sympathetic attitude toward their limitations. Building trust, therefore, depended on finding a suitable health care professional and on making an effort to create the kind of interaction that would be consistent with ongoing trust in the relationship.

Conditions for Trust

While competence and communication skills on the part of the professional, and strategic efforts on the part of the patient and family, were requisite to trusting relationships, additional conditions were also important, according to many informants. The circumstances in which their initial trust was shattered led many patients and families to question the philosophies underlying health care professionals' attitudes and the values inherent in the organization of health care delivery. They were therefore hesitant to trust health care professionals who were overly enthusiastic about the status quo or who were hooked on professional control.

In some cases, health care professionals actually helped the patients and families recognize and articulate limitations within medical science. Because such attitudes were viewed as inconsistent with traditional medical practice, they proved highly reassuring. Thus, trust was possible when the professional entertained realistic doubts about his or her expertise and that of others in the system. One woman described her frustration with a doctor whose blind spot was that he thought all doctors shared his humanitarian approach. "He thinks all other doctors are as conscientious as him, and they're not!"

A popular measure of a professional's ability to recognize flaws in the system was his or her willingness to consider alternatives. Because such therapies inherently suggested a limitation within traditional medical practice, positive attitudes toward them indicated to these informants that a professional was aware of biomedicine's limitations. Thus, ironically, the more health care professionals recognized that they could not be trusted, the easier it was for patients and families to consider them trustworthy.

Other departures from the norm of health care behavior could be similarly reassuring. For example, one woman was convinced of her physician's trustworthiness when he offered to intubate her with a pediatric nasogastric tube, rather than the adult-size one he would normally use, out of respect for her self-consciousness about her appearance. Another described a similar sense of trust associated with what she perceived as nontraditional role behaviors:

> Instead of wearing the white jacket approach, he'd come in wearing just the casual shirt and corduroy pants and moccasins, and he'd sit down. And he had a couple of easy chairs to sit in instead of, you know, technical like . . . sit in this wooden chair and I'll stand over here. So the surroundings again, and what he was wearing, and his attitude, you know . . . just gave me the feeling that he was there because he was concerned about my health.

Finally, one man expressed his doctor's departure from another unfortunate aspect of professional tradition with the following telling remark: "He never makes me feel guilty about going to see him about anything!"

In addition to departures from what these informants understood as typical health care behavior, trust required that the professional demonstrate a sense of respect for the competence and intelligence of the patient. One woman recalled the frustration of not being trusted by her physician. She said, "He wanted to deal with me as a myasthenic. I wanted to be a whole person. I don't think he was willing to trust me at all—my judgment, my feelings about things." Another expressed the frustration associated with expecting such trust from some professionals:

> We're supposed to trust her, but she has no trust of us. . . . This gets back to the whole uniqueness thing again. Quit going by the textbooks and what seems to be, and get on with finding out who these people are that you're taking care of and treat us as individuals!

In contrast, some patients and families found professionals who were willing and able to express such trust in their clients. When professionals trusted their patients, the patients found it easy to trust them in return.

> My MD now is really good that way, you know. He's excellent that way. He listens to me, what I have to say about what's wrong with me. And in

many cases, he bases his diagnosis on my contribution to it. I mean it's like
a self-diagnosis kind of thing, and he allows me to do that. And that's why
I stay with him.

Thus, an important condition for trust was that the professional trust the
patient and family. Unfortunately, many informants found this last
condition the most difficult to meet. As one commented, "That's the
only thing about the health professionals. They think that we don't use
our heads."

For those patients and families who sought trusting health care
relationships, developing and maintaining trust was a challenging proposition. Health care professionals worthy of trust had to demonstrate
some departure from expected professional attitudes or behaviors, and
had to demonstrate genuine respect for their clients' competence in
matters of chronic illness decision making. To some extent, patients and
families wanting such relationships could cultivate them with their
existing professionals; however, because there were certain conditions
under which trust was impossible, many people had to take an active
role in recruiting new professionals onto their case. For as many as were
able to create trusting relationships, there seemed an equal number who
sought one unsuccessfully. From the informants' perspective, trustworthy professionals were scarce. The wistful thoughts of one patient
illustrate:

You'd have to have a miracle mix, wouldn't you? You'd have to have a bit
of psychology, someone with miracle fingertips for a good massage,
someone who could listen and help you be a good listener too, someone
who knew all the answers. That's who you need. There's no such person.

CONFIDENT PATIENTS

Consumer and team playing relationships resulted when patients and
their families felt sufficiently confident in their own abilities to take on
the weight of responsibility for managing health care for the chronic
illness. Within the population of informants for this study, these two
relationship types were more often preferred over the long term than
were hero worship and resignation. Thus, many of the informants
described what seemed to be a "drifting to the right," along the horizontal dimension of the guarded alliance model toward increasing

confidence. This discussion will examine the nature of confidence according to the perspective of patients and families, and will consider factors that contribute to its acquisition over time.

The Value of Knowledge

In order to feel confident about their contribution to health care relationships, the patients and families required a sophisticated working knowledge of their illness and its management. This knowledge generally included pathophysiological implications of disease, current research findings and programs, the meaning of diagnostic determinants, and the range of available treatment options. Confidence with regard to such a wide variety of topics usually required extensive time in the chronic illness experience, combined with a dedication to learning. In addition, it required access to resources for developing knowledge-acquisition skills in such a specialized field.

The informants involved in this study represented backgrounds ranging from only a few years of formal education to highly educated professionals. Among the informants, there were 16 with health care professional or paraprofessional training. Further, several others were children or spouses of health care professionals. As one commented, "I guess that's partially where I get my pushiness, too. I have a lot of knowledge of the medical system through my mother." This subset of informants entered the chronic illness experience with specific knowledge and special privilege with regard to understanding the workings of the health care system. One might anticipate that their familiarity with health care language, professional distinctions, organizational structures, and biomedical theory would have eased their transition into chronicity and smoothed their health care relationships. However, their accounts demonstrated a process indistinguishable from that of the less-informed patients and families, including a naive trust and a consequent shattering of that trust.

> I think, despite the fact that I'm a nurse, I think I blindly went ahead and just accepted what people told me, and kind of expected that if we'd go in with a problem, that it would be solved, and we'd go home again and everything would be fine.

In many cases, the sense of having been betrayed by the system they thought they knew exaggerated the distress inherent in this process.

The informants who were health care professionals and paraprofessionals often reflected on the ways in which their specialized knowledge and resources might have been useful in creating a sense of confidence in their health care relationships in guarded alliance. One aspect of this confidence was the advantage it provided them in accessing information about their health condition. For many, gaining information was a natural way to respond to the crisis. As one parent explained, "My response to the stress, and also my absolutely being aghast that my child had asthma, was to do what I do with a lot of things that I'm unsure of, which was to head to the library quick." However, access to technical and medical information could be a mixed blessing, as one woman's comments illustrate: "I think having my background, that's when you dive into the books, and you start questioning the people you know, and you start finding out a little bit of knowledge is a dangerous thing." In many cases, the most immediately available information could be dangerously outdated: "Of course, I was in my books in 2 minutes, you know, looking. And my books were all out of nursing school in the early sixties, and there wasn't a whole lot on regional ileitis, let me tell you!"

Thus information, highly valued by most patients and families, seemed immediately available to those with health care professional backgrounds. Paradoxically, however, the sources to which these individuals had access were rarely the most useful. One woman reported that awareness of her nursing background caused others in her patient support group to seek her out as an information resource. When asked where she got information, however, she confessed that it came from "other MS patients and my own experiences." So learning about chronic illness involved considerably more than a professional background could provide.

For many health professionals in the informant group, their personal experience of receiving care for chronic illness seemed far removed from health care as they knew it. One woman's comments illustrate: "Certainly working in the medical world . . . didn't help me with this experience. Because it was contrary to it. . . . It seemed to be very removed from medicine as I knew it." Many found that their chronic illness experience forced them to consider healing methods and therapeutic techniques they would have considered quackery prior to this involvement.

So at this point I felt like I will try anything. Conventional or not, I will try anything. Because up to that point, you know, with this medical background, you just kind of turn your nose up at anything that isn't accepted.

Often, this experiential difference extended to the role expectations of their own profession. One nurse, for example, was shocked to discover the lack of professionalism among other nurses: "That's what makes me mad, because I understand the family's side of it, but a lot of the nurses don't understand the family's side." Observations of a quality of professional care that was substantially lower than their own would have been were particularly disturbing. As one nurse remarked, "I said to myself, 'If I ever treat a patient like they're treating me—somebody shoot me.'" The experience of obtaining health care for chronic illness shook these informants' confidence in their professions as much as it provided them with confidence in managing health care.

In some cases, health professional backgrounds offered the informants direct access to supports or services not as easily available to others. For example, one woman thought that her doctor was more forthcoming with information because of her professional status.

> He knows I'm a nurse. I've worked with him at the hospital. And I think that sometimes he may open up to me a little more because I'm not intimidated by him, where some of his patients are. And he has expressed that to me, you know.

Another used professional networks to advantage in helping her select an appropriate doctor. In other cases, these informants predicted that knowledge of their professional background might prove a liability. One woman explained how her professional status complicated the process of obtaining useful information from her doctor.

> I had the beginning stages of physiology and anatomy, and I basically know how the body functions, the joints and the bones, and what would be regular, and what wouldn't be regular (*pause*). A lot of doctors almost resent that. If you sound like, you know, "Well, I understand what you're saying." "Well, do you? This is how the body works." And they put you really back at layman's terms. . . . They obviously do resent that you might know something.

Another believed that her professional status made health care professionals more suspicious of her.

> It was fascinating that everybody knew that I was a nurse, when I would come in. . . . I know when I've visited him in the hospital, every single person from the floor cleaner to the students to the whatever says, "Oh, I understand you're a nursing instructor." And I have visions they must put the bloody (*laugh*), you know, thing all over the chart in red!

Accordingly, many of those with health care backgrounds learned to judge when to use their status to advantage and when to hide it. One nurse, for example, explained that she usually tried to play down her professional status, "but if there's a problem with [my child]'s care, then I start playing it up a little bit, because, ultimately, the reason she's there is to get better."

Therefore, being informed about health care through a professional or occupational involvement in it contributed little to a sense of confidence in handling health care relationships. The accounts of this special subset of informants reveal that the knowledge that is associated with having professional education was only marginally advantageous in the real world of coping with chronic illness. Further, they illustrate that exceptional access to the inner workings of the health care organizational structure afforded these patients and families some advantages, but perhaps an equal number of disadvantages, in negotiating for care within that system. The knowledge and skill associated with developing confidence in health care relationships, therefore, seems highly specialized to the chronic illness experience. How it is developed and maintained will now be considered.

Accepting Responsibility

As has been suggested earlier, a central element in the process of developing confidence is the shift of responsibility for health care away from the professional health care provider and toward the patient and family. Accepting responsibility for such an burden requires a reevaluation of the competencies of both the professionals and the patients and families.

According to these informants, this shift in responsibility was made possible by the realization that health care professionals were not going to fix the chronic health problem. As one man explained:

> After all, a doctor can't heal you. It's your own system that has got to do the healing, and a doctor may be able to suggest something which will help your system to heal itself but he can't heal it. He's not God Almighty.

Many of these patients and families began to believe that the confidence expressed by professionals about chronic illness management was far more bluff than substance. Specifically, they began to understand that it reflected an expertise with academic knowledge that did not prepare one for the realities of living with a chronic condition.

> He's opinionated and it shows. . . . You know he feels that his ways of doing things are right. And they probably are, but there has to be exceptions and he can't deal with any exceptions. . . . And you have to realize that people are human and there's gonna have to be exceptions.

The realization that the health care professionals were incapable of taking on full responsibility for health care in chronic illness was an important step in helping patients and families accept that responsibility themselves. However, accepting responsibility also required that patients and families reexamine their own competencies, as one woman explained:

> You have to own the problem. You can't give it to somebody else and expect them to do it. But you can get both help and advice and information in there, and at some point you will either respect it or reject it.

In this manner, the patients and families began to realize that no one knew their experience better than themselves and, as such, they had become the experts.

In some circumstances, patients and families found that accepting responsibility was more than they could manage. Such circumstances usually included either exhaustion or acuity, and afforded even the most competent of chronically ill people a release from the burden of health care decision making. Because a considerable energy expenditure was required to maintain responsibility for health care decisions, there were instances in which a shift toward placing trust in a professional was a welcome relief for these patients and families. As one woman explained, "Really, what you want is someone to come up and say, 'It's okay, you don't have to be strong anymore,' you know." Another made a similar observation:

> You know, the pressure builds up on you, and you think, "My God, why do I have to be the one that's making all of these decisions," you know. "Why doesn't somebody else just take it out of my hands," you know, "and do it for me?"

So confidence within health care relationships could be jeopardized by circumstances that reduced the informants' energy level or their knowledge with regard to the decisions at hand. Since chronic illness was rarely stable, maintaining confidence was difficult. The degree to which they were willing or able to accept responsibility for the direction of their health care was therefore critical in determining the confidence that these patients and families brought to the health care encounter.

Gaining Confidence

Because relationships characterized by confident involvement of the patient and family were highly valued by many of the informants, the accounts revealed a number of strategies by which such confidence was attained over time. In the previous discussion, this confidence has been linked to both knowledge and responsibility. How these people actually set about acquiring these will be dealt with here.

One important factor influencing the development of confidence was success in health care decision making. Therefore, those patients and families who had suffered untoward consequences from unfortunate decisions found it quite difficult to trust their judgment when it conflicted with that of a health care professional. Conversely, those who had benefited from decisions made on their own behalf found it much easier to feel confident about their judgments. As one patient remarked, "I do know what I'm doing. I've been doing the best I can for all these years, and I do know a lot."

Upon realization that much of the critical information was neither in the textbooks nor forthcoming from the professionals, many patients and families mobilized outside resources to help them make sound decisions about their situation. Some made use of multiple health care relationships to validate their interpretations and conclusions. As one woman said, "You don't learn anything from the doctors. You have to align yourself with the nursing staff." Many developed skills in using medical libraries and evaluating research reports in their efforts to make their own decisions about illness management. From an informed position, they felt more comfortable interpreting the professionals' perspective of their case. Several of these individuals had extended their quest for outside information to include contacting internationally recognized experts on the subject of their disease, and attending professional conferences.

For most of those interviewed, the most valuable resource used in this regard was the patient or family support group. From the extensive descriptions, it was evident that they offered a goldmine of relevant information about which health care professionals could be trusted, which services ought to be considered, and how to manipulate the professionals to obtain such services. As a result, the lay support group provided expert advice in ways of managing health care relationships and helped people become more confident in their abilities with health care decision making.

Another confidence-building strategy described often by these patients and families was the development of skills to advocate or "run interference" on their own behalf, as one man explained:

> Well, for me it's always been a case of the squeaky wheel gets the grease. I mean, if you scream loud enough, and keep going back to the doctor, they're going to do something, if for no other reason than to get rid of you!

Many of the informants expressed the view that speaking up on their own behalf was an essential survival skill in the context of chronic illness. As one woman claimed, "Even the really wonderful people don't respond unless you go after them often."

In some cases, the informants pointed out the advantages of learning to be confrontational and aggressive in health care relationships, as one man explained:

> You learn, not only with a chronic illness but if somebody's ill for a long time, that you have to be aggressive with the doctors. The nurses will be helpful as much as they can, and the dietitians, and the entire support staff. . . . But I found out that you really have to ask for it, you know, you put your foot down in order to get some answers.

Often this advocacy on their own behalf included lodging complaints and expressing their criticisms openly. Further, some patients and families believed that outright intimidation tactics were occasionally justifiable. One woman described such a circumstance this way: "Well, it took a tantrum or two from me then to really lay it out in spades with the guy . . . essentially because I embarrassed him with his ineffectiveness." Those who described themselves as aggressive or confrontational often expressed empathy for the health care professionals on the receiving end of their behavior, as one woman's comments illustrate: "I'm sure that she sees me as an awkward person, really, because in a sense she can't control me. And I haggle, you know, for the things that I want."

In general, the strategy of self-advocacy reflected a desire on the part of patients and families to protect their interests and obtain the help they needed. As such, it required a sophisticated analysis of the health care scene as well as a sense of confidence in their ability to make relevant judgments about their needs.

For some people, a developing sense of confidence was actually encouraged by health care professionals. In fact, some recalled how health care professionals had taught them to believe in their own abilities, as one patient's experience illustrates:

> By and large now, I've got a sense of myself. My G.P. helped me do that—that I am the best determiner of what's wrong with me, and how to deal with it. . . . It's almost like I'm going in for concurrence rather than diagnosis.

Similarly, one woman summarized her physician's guidance this way, "He is in fact giving me a sense of responsibility. He's not trying to be my father, or my protector, or anything else." When this type of encouragement occurred, the patients and families invariably viewed these health care providers as among the most enlightened of their profession. Regardless of whether they sought a trusting relationship, these people recognized such departures from traditional paternalism as evidence of that professional's trustworthiness.

The final common strategy used by many patients and families to generate confidence in their own capability was the development of a healthy skepticism toward the health care system overall. Such an attitude was expressed as the polar opposite to naive trust. As one woman recalled, "Well, going back to the beginning, it was blind trust—blind trust in all of these people who knew so much—and total faith. And now it's total skepticism." From the stance of skepticism, these patients and families were able to exercise control by selecting when and how to cooperate with their professional health care providers. As one explained, the onus was now on the health care professionals to prove their trustworthiness. "I think I have a totally negative attitude when it comes to the medical profession. Now I need it [trust] proven to me."

So the attitude of skepticism served as a paradoxical strategy for building confidence in health care relationships; by denying the possibility of trust in the existing system, patients and families felt more secure in defining exceptions to the rule. As one woman commented, "You learn to sort out the garbage from what you really need to be listening to." In addition, this skepticism served to reinforce their confidence in their own illness management. One patient articulated such an attitude this way:

> It's nice to know that there's a healthy cynicism, if you will, that will push people toward finding the best health care for them. Because I really believe that people have to invest their own energies and themselves in making themselves feel better. And what we often do to ourselves mentally and emotionally, we fail to do for ourselves physically, because we just have blind trust.

Thus the accounts of these informants explained how chronically ill individuals and their families become confident in their abilities to participate actively in their own health care, and therefore take on greater control within their health care relationships.

CONCLUSIONS

The accounts of trust and confidence in health care relationships reveal some interesting conclusions about how chronically ill people and their families understand their role in ongoing health care relationships in chronic illness. Primarily, they express the opinion that most health care professionals are not trustworthy, according to the requirements of managing a chronic health problem. Further, they explain that, from the patient's and family's perspective, trust is not always desirable. Because it can represent a position of weakness within the system, some chronically ill people and their families may be reluctant to place their trust in any professional, no matter how trustworthy.

Further, the accounts reveal that competence is important to patients and families, but is quite insufficient to permit trust. From their perspective, the competencies of a professional are relevant only if actually applied, and such application is often dependent upon such variables as whether the professional is interested in their particular case. Communication skills are also of concern to these chronically ill patients and families. However, excellence in communication is insufficient evidence that a professional ought to be trusted. Instead, the abilities to respect their patients and to recognize limitations in their own expertise seem more relevant criteria for trustworthiness from the patient's and family's perspective (Thorne & Robinson, 1988c).

The accounts also explain the role of patient confidence in managing health care relationships. The evidence provided by informants who were health care professionals as well as patients reveals that medical knowledge and familiarity with the health care system are far less relevant than is personal experiential knowledge in developing a sense of confidence in chronic illness management. Confidence also requires a major shift in responsibility for health care decisions from the professional to the patient and family. While both failures in the health care arena and the patient's growing information base facilitate this transition, the weight of responsibility may be too great a burden in some cases. Thus, confidence in health care relationships involves considerable commitment.

Finally, the accounts reveal the extent to which both trust and confidence depend on a growing skepticism about the larger picture in health care. Because they have analyzed the health care system's response to chronic illness and found it lacking, these patients and families challenge us to interpret their health care relationships within that larger domain. From their perspective, successful relationships that include trust or confidence are possible only when the norms of typical health care professional behavior are violated. Thus, they invite us to further our consideration of such relationships on the basis of a critical analysis of the nature of health care in our society, the way the health care system influences health care professionals, and, finally, the way it shapes the experience of those who are chronically ill.

PART THREE

The Institutional Experience

SEVEN

Confrontations With the
Health Care System

While relationships with individual health care professionals caused consternation among the chronically ill individuals and their families in this study, encounters with the health care system as a whole resembled a head-on collision. In this final set of chapters, the chronic illness experience will be examined at the most global level of analysis—the interaction between individuals, their relationships, and the systems in which they converge. Through an exploration of how the health care system appears to those who become involved in it by virtue of a chronic illness experience, a unique perspective on the current problems in health care will be articulated.

Earlier chapters have addressed some of the particularly challenging aspects of life with a chronic health problem. They have peered into the accounts of individual lives and have searched out common ground in the journey into chronicity. They have also explored the social climate within which a chronic illness is understood in today's modern world. Extending the inquiry into the social dynamics that shape chronic illness, a second set of chapters has examined the relationships within which the primary transactions of chronic illness are conducted. Using the perspective of patients and families as its foundation, this discussion illuminated the power and authority of such health care relationships in shaping critical dimensions in the lives of those who are ill. Further, this discussion challenged us to deepen our analysis in an effort to make sense of what it is that makes relationships in health care so tortured and so tenuous. What is this system, if not the individuals within it?

This chapter will begin this final set of analyses by exploring the accounts of something that chronically ill patients and their families came to call "the system." As one man explained, nothing in their past experience had prepared them for this particular confrontation, an encounter so profound that it would influence their understanding of the world from this point forward.

> I mean, you don't really think of the system when you're looking for immediate treatment. . . . You don't even think about it in terms of individuals of the system. But, when you start hitting points of frustration, then you start. Then the analysis comes in.

In this chapter, two general categories of confrontations will provide the focus of discussion; those having to do with the organizational structure of health care, and those having to do with the way in which human beings conduct themselves within that structure. Following this discussion, two subsequent chapters will document the response of chronically ill people and their families to the organizational and sociocultural battles they find themselves engaged in. The analysis will finally conclude with a chapter exploring changes that would be necessary for any meaningful solution to the problems of the chronically ill in the existing health care system.

ORGANIZATIONAL ISSUES

As has become evident through the accounts thus far, the bureaucratic structure of health care was of concern to the chronically ill and their families. Although few had given health care organization and delivery much thought prior to their own personal encounter with chronic illness, most came to appreciate its intricate complexities with increasing sophistication over time. Their preoccupation with it reflected the extent to which it impinged on their lives and alerted them to its relevance in the chronic illness story.

In this discussion, four impressions of the organizational structure will be described. Each represents one dimension of a complex social institution whose full dimensions were never completely revealed to any one individual. Thus, a portrait of "the system" will be generated via the technique of drawing together common elements through the special angle from which each informant formed his or her ideas. In this way, the accounts create a composite portrait of the chronic illness perspective of what it is like to obtain health care.

Falling Through the Cracks

In contrast to the organ transplant patients featured in the tabloids, for whom no expense was too great, and toward whose recovery teams of highly trained professionals eagerly invest all the time, energy, and goodwill at their disposal, the overriding interpretation of the chronically ill was that they had somehow fallen through the cracks of the health care system. For their life-and-death issues, there was relatively little money, energy, or sympathy forthcoming from anyone either inside or outside the system. Those who had previous experience with a dramatic acute illness in themselves or in a close family member were often astounded at the differential treatment that the chronically ill experienced within the same health care system.

In spite of the fact that there was no available cure and often limited available treatments, many chronically ill people found themselves swept into a whirlwind of health care involvement. The story of Rowena, a middle-aged woman with arthritis, captures such an experience so graphically that it will be offered here in some detail. Rowena's first rheumatologist told her she didn't have arthritis. Then, "I got one that they said was the brain of the institute. And a little cockier man I've never met." After a thorough examination, he put Rowena on a medication, and asked her to return in 2 months for tests. In that 2 months, she lost her hearing almost completely. On the advice of an ear specialist, she went off the medication, and her hearing returned. When she returned to the rheumatologist, he confirmed her serious case of rheumatoid arthritis, and asked her to double her dose of the medication. She protested, and he was furious, telling her there was no relationship between the medication and her hearing problem. Two years later, Rowena was referred to a third rheumatologist. This one was a highly respected young woman, but far too busy with a new baby at home to be available to her patients. "And there was me thinking, 'Well, gosh, number three! What's wrong with me?' But each thing was something a little different." A fourth rheumatologist, who entered the scene when she was admitted to a rehabilitation center for inpatient therapy, was interested in performing every imaginable blood test. "I began to get paranoid about my blood tests, and then she started zeroing in on that paranoia." One day, this rheumatologist held a staff conference at which Rowena was the focus of discussion.

> It feels more like an inquisition than a conference. Especially when they set you up, you know, you're sort of up on a platform so they can all see

you. . . . She chose that one day to sort of tell everybody, you know, that I had this phobia about blood tests, and that she thought I should go to the phobia clinic, and get over it, before she could advance further. . . . I felt like she was belittling me in front of all those people.

Following this hospitalization, she was referred to a fifth rheumatologist by a nurse at the arthritis clinic. After seeing her only once, he referred Rowena to a sixth the following year. This one thought she was a candidate for hand, knee, and hip surgeries, so had her admitted to another rehabilitation center, where she encountered her seventh rheumatologist.

I liked him. I liked his attitude. . . . But then the very day that you left [the center] you left him completely and that was it. There was no nothing. . . . I guess they can't get too involved intimately. They keep saying that your family doctor is the one to talk to, and my family doctor retired while I was in there.

As her story continued, Rowena had subsequent encounters with rheumatologists number three and five, but was unable to develop any functional relationship with either. Her inability to find a place for herself within the system was a source of deep distress, and she ruminated about the wisdom of choices she had made along the way.

Then, as I look back over it all, I keep thinking, when I try to tell somebody what has happened, like I have related to you this morning, it sounded to me like I was being a complainer and that a person who would be hearing that would think, "Good Lord," you know, if it was a new person they were meeting, and I'm not sure I want this person as a patient because nothing goes right for her. So I felt that maybe I'd better work it through myself so that nobody would have to say that.

Two and a half years after she was first interviewed, Rowena had become quite philosophical about her experience.

I thought I would be a rheumatologist in my next life because it was a cinch job (*laugh*) . . . because when you go to them and say you have an ache or a pain or something that, you know, really you want them to talk to you about it a bit—they sort of tell you, "Well, that's to be expected."

Like so many others, this woman certainly had theoretical access to health care but was unable to find the support or assistance she needed within the system. While she was able to get appointments with individual professionals, each one had an idea of his or her role that was incompatible with this patient's needs. Another patient interpreted the basic problem:

> You get the royal runaround (*laugh*) in the sense that—"Well, I've done everything that I know. These don't seem to work. Go to the next department." The next department says, "Well, we don't really treat your type, but I'll take a look at you to see what I can tell you." And they tell you the exact same thing. You often wonder if they just read your paper and just tell you what you already know.

As a result, many people found themselves in a revolving door of specialists and services without anyone willing to make a commitment.

Because no individual professional considered himself or herself their primary resource, many patients and families felt adrift and alone in a frustrating situation. Often, they discovered information and resources to which they were entitled quite by accident. For example, one woman learned from another patient that the $400 per month she spent on sterile catheters for intermittent urinary drainage was unnecessary because her catheters could easily be resterilized at home for free. Another learned from two pharmacy students assigned to interview her for a term paper that her persistent insomnia was a side effect of her current medications. At times such as these, patients and families despaired because of a system in which no one took the time to help them make sense of it all.

Adding to the frustration was their belief that professionals were reaping significant financial benefit from their illness without actually providing any valuable service. One woman described such frustration with a dermatologist involved in her care:

> I don't know what he collected every 3 weeks for walking into his office. And he would look at it and say, "Oh, they're doing fine and they're clean." And you'd wrap them up again, and that was it. You just went there every 2 to 3 weeks and they looked at them. And to me this is what makes health care so expensive. . . . It's very wrong!

Another informant deeply resented professionals being paid salaries for providing what they thought ought to be given, rather than what the chronically ill person actually required.

She came out to the house, and she said, "Don't worry, Mrs. R. When you need a wheelchair, we'll get you one." This was my introduction to MS. They started to turn me into a cripple! . . . And she's gonna sit in her cushy office down there, earning about $40,000 a year, just talking to new patients, and telling them that they'll get a wheelchair when they need one. I see through all that. I do. Something has to be done!

Thus the rewards of participating in a whirlwind of health care were hardly equivalent to the effort expended in many cases.

Another way in which many people fell between the cracks was by failing to conform to a standardized set of expectations about their needs. For example, one woman recalled an encounter in which a health care professional was so focused on a standard plan that she could not hear the patient.

She was so preprogrammed into counseling me on rejection of the wheelchair that she didn't hear what I was saying to her. I was sharing experiences with her, tongue-in-cheek and laughing about, "Boy, they don't make the aisles wide enough." I thought I was doing pretty good, because I was able to take it in a joking manner. But every time I'd say something, she'd come back with this, like I say, the counseling for rejection. I was so frustrated that day by the time she left, I was just beside myself, because she never heard me.

Even when the cracks were acknowledged by all concerned, patients and their families could still fall in, as one father's experience illustrates. Following a case conference ("I call it the $3,000-an-hour meeting, because of the professions that were involved"), the only decision was that nothing could be done because the case fell between the mandates of various government ministries. Another problem described by some patients and families was the assumption that all health care in chronic illness ought to take place during standard business hours, a time during which many struggled to maintain careers and education. Thus, standardized services rarely matched the timing and uniqueness of each patient's and family's needs.

In spite of the fact that all of the patients and families in this study lived in a country that provides health insurance and equal access to services, many found that there were serious gaps regarding which services were provided. Further, these patients and families often found what they considered to be alarming inequities within the system. For example, one woman noticed that the best equipped handicapped children were always foster children.

What those foster children need they get from the government—and nothing but the best quality! What makes those two kids any better than my child? I'm not saying they're any less of a child than my child, either, but what makes them that much better than my child? Plus, she's making a living looking after those kids. They get paid over a grand a child per month! Why can't I have something for looking after my own child then? I don't even want the thousand, I'll settle for 50 to 100 bucks a month, you know. I mean, I should just give him up and go turn around and foster my own child back and I'd get paid back—and make a hell of a good living out of it. This system is all wrong. It's almost like they encourage you to give up your kids.

Because this family was struggling with serious financial problems, the inequity was especially frustrating. From their point of view, their willingness to raise their own child further handicapped him in his ability to achieve health. As the father pointed out, their family stability deprived their child of health care.

We even thought about that at one point. We said, "Why don't I take off this weekend, and then Monday morning you can go to Welfare and say your husband has buggered off. And you'll get all kinds of things." But, you know, I hate doing that. I wouldn't do that, because, you know, we started as a family and hopefully we'll end as one—and [our son]'s a part of it, and that's the way it is. So we'll just stick together and just do whatever we have to do. It's too bad there isn't more.

In this manner, patients and families defined their health care needs in a way that departed quite considerably from the health services deemed essential by the health insurance scheme.

As has been described in an earlier chapter on acute episodes within chronic illness, hospitalizations were often mentioned as a time in which patients and their families slipped through the cracks of the system. One gentleman's humiliating experience illustrates:

And then I had to, of course, ask for assistance to be put on the commode. And that's not always the easiest thing because you had to find an orderly and then you have to have two nurses, and I have to be physically lifted from the bed and planted on this commode. And then of course once you're on the commode, and God knows where everybody's gone, but I've long finished my little job and I'm looking and waiting, and hoping and wondering. And pretty soon visiting hours come. There was one day in the afternoon, it was after 2 o'clock—well, I had been put on to the commode around 1 o'clock, and I was still sitting on the darn commode when I had a chum of mine come to visit, and all the while he was there I was sitting on this commode talking to him . . . I was there at least probably two and a half hours anyway sitting on that commode. There was nobody around to ask for help.

Often, they found themselves ignored because their problems were not sufficiently dramatic to attract the attention of hospital staff. As one man explained, "They were busy, busy people who could only spare a few minutes for you because they had a million other lives to save that afternoon." Thus, hospitalization provoked many of the most frustrating health care confrontations for these patients and families.

According to these informants, chronically ill people could become lost in the system very easily. So they were tempted to wonder what the system was really for if not for sick people. As one man put it, "You know, they want the ideal system where they can go about their work with absolutely nothing to get in their way." Falling through the cracks, therefore, seemed an inevitable consequence of having a health problem that the system really wasn't interested in solving.

Being a Guinea Pig

A second organizational issue that confronted the chronically ill patients and families was the health care system's expectation that they would willingly contribute to medical research and education. By virtue of their frequent involvement with health care services, they were easy prey for practicing students and eager researchers. In principle, none objected; in practice, however, their experiences sometimes confirmed their suspicions that their part in the system was merely to provide the raw materials.

Many patients and families obtained their most specialized medical assessments from physicians who were also medical professors. Consequently, although they had access to the brightest and the best, or at least that's what everyone reassured them, there was little opportunity for interaction. One woman recalled such an experience:

Dr. D. would come through with his trailings of people that were learning to be specialists. And they all examined me, three or four of them. And I have nothing against that, because I realize they have to learn, too, but each one of them examines you, and then he examines you, and then you hear them out in the hall discussing your case. Well, nobody tells me anything. You just lay there and wonder what's gonna happen now?

Another reflected on the primary motive for such encounters. "You always felt that the primary reason for your being there was for him to lecture." Similarly, one young woman recalled being told that a professional would take her case only if she agreed to be filmed for educational purposes. Another contribution to teaching included participating in endless interviews for the purpose of obtaining case histories. Given the complexity of many of their medical histories, many found it unduly frustrating to be expected to memorize and repeat all the details to each new student or practitioner.

> I hate all this case history stuff, you know. We've been in hospital three times, and I know it's a teaching hospital, and I know it gives practice to these people, and so therefore I do it. But . . . I don't want to tell the story of [my son] again, you know. Like, "Read it," you know. It's there.

Although frustrated with students, most people did not believe they had the right to refuse. "I was also asked to have other students—medical students. When I had said no, I got persuaded." In other cases, patients were never asked about their willingness to be the lesson of the day.

> The doctor in charge of the emergency was doing the rounds with the medical students, and he walked up to my bed and spoke about me in the third person. And I kept on trying to interrupt him and ask him things. I may as well have not been there. That again was one of the more uncanny experiences I ever have had. I was not there. It was a case, and they didn't even look at me. They looked right through me. To this very day, I can visualize them standing there. And they just walked on to the next bed. No one said anything.

Further, they sometimes felt completely misled about the role they were playing in medical education. One woman, for example, recalled her shock at seeing her son's cardiac surgeon in the hospital cafeteria while the operation was actually in progress. On inquiry, she was told that students and residents were performing the operation and that the surgeon would look in on them later.

The other subtle expectation faced by these patients and families was that they make themselves available to whatever research was in progress. Because they saw medical research as their hope for the future, most were eager to volunteer to be subjects for anything that might lead to an effective treatment or intervention. However, many found that they were often excluded from active participation by what they thought to be arbitrary or unnecessarily harsh exclusion criteria. For example, one woman discovered that the potential risks precluded human testing of the only promising treatment available for her condition.

> The only drawback was, a few of [the mice] died. Now, the way this is, you either get really better or you die (*laugh*). At the gathering 'round the table, everybody's thinking, "So what?" you know, "I'll take my chances." Everybody was talking about it. They're willing to try it, right? Who wants to just sit and watch game shows when you got a chance to either really live, or get it over with. And the percentage of dying was so small that it's not bad. Then I find it's gonna be another 5 years! They got the AMA and the FDA and the XYZ, and it goes on and on, all this bureaucratic red tape, and the double blind this, and the double blind that. And half the people I know won't even be around to hear the results.

From their point of view, then, there were logical and ethical flaws in the research game.

Beyond actually volunteering, many patients and families found themselves inadvertent research subjects due to the health care system's expectations that they subject themselves to any tests that the professionals suggested. One woman recalled such an instance:

> I had one doctor, who I didn't even know, who took me out for tests. He was a pathologist who had an interest in Myasthenia, and I was the only one around with it. When he found out I was in, he wanted to do an EMG test on me, which is a diagnostic test. And was unnecessary because I'd been diagnosed, and it was horrendous! I mean, these are electrical currents shooting through you like crazy. No one told me I was going to have it done. My doctor didn't authorize it. This guy just did it. I came back from that test—I was in tears. I mean, the pain was unbelievable, he was just shooting it through like crazy. Oh, God. And when I found out that my doctor had nothing to do with it, I was just furious!

Another form of such testing included participating in consultations with experts in the field. As many informants discovered, each specialist required a fixed battery of diagnostic procedures, many of which were painful, humiliating, or dangerous. Because, from the patient's and family's perspective, such extensive testing was justifiable only if the purpose was either diagnosis or prescribing treatment, many were eventually convinced that the consultation system was set up for the purpose of allowing specialists complete access to research data. As one woman commented, "Actually, it makes me kind of mad, 'cause we're guinea-pigs. . . . If we don't offer to go in, and do these things, what's going to happen?"

Further, many people reported instances in which they actually felt coerced into being research subjects if they wished ongoing treatment. One woman recalled such an experience:

> I was told I was given a choice, and all I could see was an ultimatum. [The doctor] was participating in what a pharmaceutical company wanted to do in terms of marketing its product. So therefore, there was a conflict of interest. It was not a legitimate piece of research in comparing one drug against another . . . and it was biased from the start, because a pharmaceutical company had a vested interest. . . . To see myself violated in that way—that, for me, was very unforgivable. And particularly when the staff, and the head of the ward, also saw me as being wrong to question the doctor. And that I was creating waves, and upsetting her staff, and splitting her staff, some wanting to agree with me, and others wanting to agree with the doctor, and others having nothing to say.

Like many others, this woman was under the distinct impression that health care was used as the dangling carrot to encourage research subjects. Thus, being a research subject was often understood as the currency with which health care was negotiated. Clearly, for the chronically ill and their families, the system saw them as guinea pigs in professional education and research.

Suffering Incompetence

The third category of organizational confrontations described by the informants in this study reflected their perceived vulnerability to all manner of error and incompetence within the system. While there was some opportunity for the chronically ill and their families to shop for competence in their primary health care relationships, there was often little that could be done to protect them from the possibility of incompetence in many other arenas of health care. Frequent hospitalizations, diagnostic testing, home support services, or ongoing therapies brought many of the chronically ill into close contact with a variety of workers over whom they had little control, and a range of services into which they had little input. They perceived themselves as particularly vulnerable to acts of incompetence and human error. The accounts illustrate the horror, fear, and frustration that perceived incompetence generated in those living with chronic illness.

Sprinkled among the accounts were a litany of outright errors from the perspective of the chronically ill individuals and families. One woman recalled a stress test in which the technician set the machine at a level that might have killed a less assertive cardiac patient than her husband. Another recalled a hospital dietitian providing her with a typed copy of a diet that could have endangered her life, had she followed it at home. Recognizing the error the next day, the dietitian telephoned the patient and offered to put the correct diet in the mail, but offered no information as to what the woman was to eat in the interim. Other patients and families reported incorrect interpretation of X-rays or other tests, sometimes leading to misdiagnoses or unnecessary surgeries; required medications withheld or incorrect ones given in error; and inappropriately applied treatments and therapies.

In many cases, these informants were on the receiving end of serious acts of incompetence. For example, one patient recalled an occasion on which his Stryker frame was turned without the safety equipment fastened. "It was like hell. It was incredible. . . . I got whipped back down to surgery . . . and I didn't wake up again for about 4 days." Another recalled the ineptitude of one particular intravenous nurse:

> She'd go in to get the vein, and she'd miss, and then she started moving it around, and jabbing, and she'd never get anywhere, so she'd pull it out, and she'd try somewhere else. . . . I think she tried nine times on me in a row.

Similarly, a third reported incompetence on the part of a physician:

> I guess it was a young anesthetist, and he thought I looked super healthy . . . I guess he didn't read my chart that closely to see my history. . . . So he didn't bother to intubate me during the operation. So naturally . . . I aspirated and developed pneumonia.

In many cases, the incompetence was complicated by an utter unwillingness to listen to the patient or family's warnings.

> As soon as the dye went in the vein I went into a crisis situation. . . . That was just an automatic reaction. He wouldn't listen to me when I was trying to tell him. He came with the Demerol, he shot me through with Demerol, and the nurse noticed that I had stopped breathing, and she did CPR (cardiopulmonary resuscitation). And at the end of that, I said, "From now on, I want control."

Being hospitalized also subjected patients and their families to observations of what they considered incompetent care of other patients. One informant recalled his horror when a nurse insisted that his elderly roommate with a cardiac problem take a shower, despite being on full bed rest. When the gentleman died in the shower, the patient was convinced that the nurse had killed him. Similarly, a young man described an incident in which he was unable to obtain help for a roommate who was falling out of bed:

> I could hear all the nurses at the nurses station talking, giggling, and laughing, and all that stuff, and I pushed the button. And I couldn't do a thing. . . . It took almost a half an hour for them to get in there, and here [the roommate] was holding on for dear life on those rails. And the only reason they finally came in is I got—I started calling them every name in the book . . . and they finally came in to tell me to shut up. The guy had a hip replacement yesterday, he's falling out of bed, and you dumb bitches can't even come in here and get him back into bed. And he was screaming his head off too. . . . Just incredible!

Being witness to what they interpreted as incompetence in the care of others was terrifying for many patients and families.

While the life-and-death errors were obviously the most dramatic, many of the chronically ill patients and families were also concerned about the degree of minor error that was tolerated in general health care practice. One aspect of professional health care that concerned them in this way was the standardization of treatments and procedures. As one woman noticed, many professionals were insistent on going by the book, even when it defied logic. "Like, I weigh 103, and they might tell a 200-pound man the same thing. It doesn't make sense." Another woman experienced a disastrous outcome from a standard physical therapy procedure. Because her chronic illness had weakened the surrounding musculature, the procedure dislocated her hip and caused permanent soft tissue damage. From the perspective of patients and families, competence was not simply a matter of knowing and following standard procedures, but also, and more important, a matter of common sense.

The question of competence also arose when patients and families were given conflicting advice by equally expert health care professionals, as one woman explained:

> Each doctor has a different opinion. The surgeon . . . that did the bypass said, "Oh, there's nothing wrong with you now. You're fine. . . . You can

eat anything you want." And yet, when I talked to my own family physician he said, "Oh, no, it's not so. You must stay on a diet." . . . So there's a difference between a surgeon and my own family physician. . . . I mean, who do you believe?

Similarly, many were shocked to experience conflicting opinions within an individual professional.

I'm sitting there in so much pain I can't see straight. So then, believe it or not, he booked me back into the hospital. . . . I remember they put the IV (intravenous) in me, because I was supposed to be going for surgery. He comes in like, no kidding, 15 minutes before I'm supposed to go down, and he says, "I'm sorry, but I don't know what I'm doing." That's what he said to me! So out comes the IV, and off I go home. I couldn't believe it.

Such errors inevitably produced anxious responses in both patients and families.

For many of the chronically ill individuals and families in this study, incompetence had a profound effect on their quality of life with chronic illness. Several were certain that their symptoms would have been manageable had they received appropriate intervention early in their illness. However, in most cases, the acts they considered incompetent were not regarded as such within the medical establishment. Further, these patients and families were rarely satisfied that the same acts of incompetence would not be repeated on future patients.

The horror of having witnessed or been party to an act that they considered incompetent was compounded by the inability of the patients and families to do anything to rectify the situation. From their perspective, incompetence within the health care system was a serious problem and a major threat to the safety and well-being of chronically ill patients.

Getting Caught in Red Tape

The final category of organizational difficulty that characterized health care for these chronically ill individuals and families was the regulations within health care delivery. As these people discovered, it was very difficult to challenge a highly bureaucratized health care system. For example, Laverne became entangled in what ought to have been a very simple referral procedure when her son developed an unusual skin lesion. Because the doctor who first spotted it was a specialist, he sent her back to her family doctor to be formally referred to a dermatologist. Despite the lengthy wait to obtain it, the formal referral never actually arrived, and Laverne had to arrange to have the family doctor's receptionist telephone the dermatologist to confirm that it had been sent. Further, she ended up having to explain the entire history herself, much to the dismay of the dermatologist. As Laverne concluded:

> Bureaucracy, you know, has caught up with them. . . . Why do three people not talk to each other (*laugh*) . . . it's so ridiculous. It's just bureaucracy overlapping each other, and catching up with its own tail, you know. It's just crazy.

In most cases, the bureaucratic requirements of health care delivery seemed predicated on completely faulty logic. For example, one woman remembered her father being shuffled back and forth through a total of six hospital wards during a single week of hospitalization. Similarly, a young man noted the nonsensical practice of requiring hospitalized patients to take sedatives at night.

> At first, they said you have to take them, 'cause they were prescribed. And [my doctor] came in . . . and she got them taken off my chart. And they'd still come down to the TV room with these stupid sleeping pills and a glass of water. I got to the point where I didn't even argue any more. . . . I'd go back in my room, and I'd hide them.

Yet another illogical aspect of the health care bureaucracy, according to the patients and families, was requiring them to come to the doctor's office for regular prescriptions or test results, rather than using the telephone. In many cases, fatigue and immobility made extra office visits extremely difficult, as one woman complained: "It's a bureaucracy, which is tiring and useless to me as a patient person. It seems like it's not pragmatic at all." In other instances, patients suspected that it was more lucrative for professionals to plan office visits than to use the telephone.

> He'd have me come in, and I would have had tests, and I would have an appointment to see him after these tests were done, and I would go in to keep that appointment, and I would wait, sometimes an hour and a half to go in for him to tell me that the results of the test weren't back yet, instead of a phone call to say, "Mrs. L., the results are—so-and-so," or "I want to

see you again so-and-so." And I got fed up with that. Like I didn't catch
on to what was happening right away.

For many patients and families, the strict rules and regulations governing home support services were unbelievably frustrating. For example, one patient discovered that the woman from a homemaker service
was forbidden to assist her with rinsing shampoo out of her hair unless
it was washed during an assisted tub bath because the service's hair-
dresser (for which she did not qualify) had a monopoly on shampoos.
From their point of view, such regulations created financial inefficiency
as well as frustration. One family's search for respite so that they could
continue to care for their chronically ill child at home was a particularly
poignant example. They discovered that while the government would
cover the high cost of institutionalizing their son, it would not reimburse
them for a babysitter once a month to preserve their struggling marriage.

> If I put him in one of those respite homes forever, you can almost guarantee
> he'll never be anything in the world. He'll always be a vegetable. And so
> it's going to keep costing the taxpayers money, and money, until the day
> he dies. But if we can get him to end up going out on his own, it's not gonna
> cost the taxpayers. That's why I just don't understand all this . . . red tape.

Another very common experience in dealing with a health care
bureaucracy was waiting. While most people were willing to tolerate
waiting if it seemed necessary, they were angry at the way many
professionals and services completely ignored the needs of patients in
their booking schemes. One man recalled discovering that there were
six others in a physician's waiting room, all scheduled in the same time
slot.

> What he would do was, he'd get through all those people in the morning,
> then he'd go out and play golf in the afternoon, you see. I know it isn't any
> of my business, but he made enough money to have worked a day and a
> half for the amount of people that he could cram in by noon.

As noted earlier, many patients and families were referred to one practitioner after another in the course of their illness. In such cases, each new
practitioner meant more waiting. The wait might lead to the discovery of
an excellent practitioner, but one to whom the patient would have restricted access, as the following account illustrates:

> They won't give you an appointment under 3 months. And you're supposed to, if there's anything happens, go and see your family doctor. . . . That bothers me . . . I'm afraid that I would get the same answer that I just got from him the other day. "I'll make that decision. I'll tell you when you need to see a specialist." They don't want to let go of that power or control or whatever it is.

Another common bureaucratic hassle described by these patients and families was the impossible challenge of trying to reach professionals by telephone.

> And you're trying to get him on the phone, and you get, "Oh, he's not in right now, and he's not very good about returning his calls." Oh, isn't that just bloody marvelous! Oh, I couldn't believe it! And then you phone in again—busy, busy. Phone in again, "Oh, he's gone for the whole month of August. You might be lucky if you phone in September."

The regulations surrounding access to professionals were a source of extreme anxiety for some people. For example, one young man recalled intense frustration in trying to find out the outcome of his wife's major surgery. Despite repeated phone calls to the hospital, the surgeon's office, and everyone else he could think of, he was unable to obtain any information, other than learning that such information would not be given out by telephone. Thus, according to many patients and families, restricted telephone access added considerably to the frustration of chronic illness.

Another frustration associated with the bureaucratic structure was dealing with the turf battles between the health care professions. Similar territorial wars were waged over which treatments and therapies would be supported by the health insurance program.

> You know, the effective treatment, they won't pay for it. My vitamins, they won't pay for it. They'll pay for me to be blitzed out of my fucking tree but they won't pay for vitamins. You know, they'll pay for me to see every fucking specialist on this earth, but they won't foot the bill for me to have a psychologist, or a psychotherapist. . . . You know, where's the justice in the fucking system?

Because the physicians typically controlled access to other aspects of the system, their position in the pecking order could be influential in a patient's illness career.

My dear old doctor retired, and to have a new young doctor with no clout is very difficult for a long-term patient (*laugh*), which I discovered. I didn't know at that time that it takes months to get referrals and hospital privileges, and all those things just aren't quite as they should be with younger doctors.

Thus, learning the politics of health care was an important part of learning the bureaucracy.

Because of standard treatment or care plans, many patients and families found that they were subject to repeated and senseless procedures, regardless of whether they needed them. As a nurse with an asthmatic child commented, "I get taught how to take her temperature every time I go." Like this woman, many of the patients and families learned to enjoy the morbid humor inherent in such bureaucratic nonsense. One man, for example, recalled an incident of bureaucratic record-keeping in the midst of what was, to him, a dire emergency:

I admitted myself in the middle of the night with a kidney stone, not knowing it was a kidney stone, never having had a kidney stone before. Not knowing, being completely in the dark about the source of this extreme pain. And of course the first person to interview me was, I guess, the third-year medical student who asked me for my name and—what else?—medical number. I babbled away something, and the next morning I looked at what I babbled away and it had no bearing on reality whatsoever. My address, my telephone, all that was fictitious. And so was the medical number. He kept on prompting me until I gave him nine digits. That was it. Believe it or not, I got my name correct.

Thus, the incredibly complex and infuriating red tape of health care affected the chronically ill and their families in many ways. At best, it was humorous and frustrating. At worst, it made rational health care an almost impossible challenge for even the best informed and the most assertive of clients.

The accounts provide a graphic portrait of a number of major problems created by the organizational structure of health care delivery. For the chronically ill and their families, the journey into health care is an odyssey of rules, regulations, and policies that make little sense and provide little obvious benefit to anyone. From their point of view, the system makes obtaining health care extremely complex and, at times, almost impossible. Further, they suspect that it represents neither a cost-effective nor a socially responsible organizational structure. Consequently, their confrontations with the organization of health care challenge them to try to make sense of the system for themselves.

SOCIOCULTURAL ISSUES

The second major category of health care system confrontations articulated by the patients and families in this study reflects their intimate encounters with the individual people that society charges with delivering health care services. Because such services are essentially human services, the behaviors and attitudes of health care workers are of considerable influence upon those whose illness is ongoing. In this discussion, a variety of unpleasantries encountered by patients and families will be reported. Clearly, not all health care encounters are unpleasant. In fact, most of the accounts in this study included vivid recollections of wonderful people and caring acts within the health care system. However, the accounts also demonstrate the power and the impact that even a single negative encounter could have on the lives and emotional states of those dealing with chronic illness. Accordingly, the sociocultural experience within the health care system represents a major source of confrontation for many chronically ill people and their families.

Prejudicial Attitudes

Like people everywhere, those who were employed in a health care capacity could be racist, sexist, homophobic, or similarly prejudiced. However, in the health context, such attitudes were particularly frightening and disturbing because they were inescapable and because they represented the antithesis of caring. Often, the prejudices were unspoken and subtle. As one Jewish man explained, "I have certain reservations, you know. If he becomes aware of our racial background, is [my wife] going to be in jeopardy?"

Although the Canadian health care system portrays itself as equally accessible to rich and poor alike, those patients and families who were not among the more privileged classes experienced considerable prejudice in their encounters with health care. As one patient pointed out, "When they find out that I'm on Welfare, it's sort of push me aside and wait in line." The daughter of another patient had a similar observation:

There is definitely, definitely a difference in the way she was treated when her address was on the west side of town, and the way that she has been

treated using our address on the east side of town (*laugh*). And I know that
is really weird, but you can just see the difference in people's reaction.

Class differences were often most apparent when home support
services of some type were required. One woman recalled "making sure
that the house was spotless" before a social worker visited for fear that
her mother might be denied home care. In other cases, the social class
of the family with chronic illness was considerably more advantaged
than that of the health care worker. One quite disabled woman, for
example, believed that the homemakers supplied by the public health
department resented her privilege.

> Like we had one lady that used to come in here. . . . She was here to do the
> vacuuming once a month, and . . . she'd walk in the house all storming all
> the time and she'd say, "I don't know why I'm here to clean your house.
> My house is way dirtier than yours, and here I am," you know. And, "My
> toilets are so filthy." And I mean, it's not my problem.

Finally, others suspected that there were disadvantages to being considered middle class, as one family member explained:

> I got the feeling sometimes that middle-class people don't need help . . .
> that if he was poorer, he would've been better off in terms of support
> systems. Which I had wondered whether a social worker would have gone
> in and seen how he was doing. Would home care have been offered? I
> almost had this feeling in a sense you were negatively penalized for being
> middle class.

Thus, many people believed that class distinctions had in some way
influenced their health care experience.

Another element of prejudice experienced by some chronically ill
individuals was the unfair assumption that they were alcoholics or drug
addicts. In some cases, aspects of their medical condition produced
signs and symptoms that were easily misinterpreted as intoxication. In
other cases, their assertiveness in trying to get their health care needs
met was misconstrued. Many patients found health care professionals
especially judgmental about their use of analgesics.

> But in the long run, you know, for somebody who's got a chronic ill-
> ness . . . so they need an extra shot for pain, that's the way they're coping,
> kind of thing, at that time. And sometimes you get some nurses—not all of

them, but some of them—where they go, "Oh, not that guy again," you know. Then they go home and instantly have a glass of wine to cope for the day that they've just had, you know.

Often, the fact that they required analgesia on a long-term basis clouded all other impressions of their health care needs. As one recalled, "I wasn't impressed with this asshole fucking doctor (*laugh*). All she could focus on me was the amount of analgesics I'm using now. . . . She's got me slotted as a drug addict." In contrast, an awareness of the social attitudes surrounding those with chemical dependencies caused some patients and families to be highly secretive about such problems. As one family member explained:

> I knew that if I wanted any really good care for her I'd better not admit to any doctor, or any health care worker, or person in the health care field, that she had ever had any problem with alcohol at all, ever.

Thus, prejudices about alcohol and drug use also influenced the health care experience of several of these informants.

Beyond racism, classism, and other common social prejudices, the chronically ill individuals and their families articulated a special brand of misapplied psychological theory they attributed to prejudice against the ill and disabled. Many found that their legitimate needs were often interpreted as neurotic. As one explained, "I seem to get the opinion from the doctor, from the nurse, from the people around there, that I am a hypochondriac." As has been noted in earlier chapters, problems for which an organic cause could not be pinpointed were generally deemed psychosomatic. One woman expressed intense frustration at what she considered an injustice: "They're not denying that my body is all fucked. They know for a fact it's fucked. And yet they tell me to investigate the psychological aspects of it, because they do not know the organic cause." Others reported being considered hysterical or neurotic because they were justifiably anxious and depressed about their escalating pain or weakness.

According to these individuals and families, many health care professionals used a limited knowledge of holistic and cross-cultural theories as yet one more assault on the credibility of their patients. For example, one woman referred to a physician's abuse of such theory:

> And then he says to me, "Well, you know, pain is all in your head. And the Chinese can walk on hot coals, and Italians they get a little sliver and they'll cry. It's all one condition." I thought, "Oh, my God."

From their perspective, psychological distress was inevitable in chronic illness. Further, most were willing to seek help for their psychological health when necessary. However, from their standpoint, popular theory about the connections between mind and body offered some unscrupulous health care workers justification for unfair biases toward the chronically ill. In this way, such theories legitimized attitudes toward patients that were as prejudicial as were classism and racism.

Power Struggles

A second category of human confrontations depicted in the accounts was the struggle for ultimate authority. Given the battle for control over decision making that has been described within the context of ongoing health care relationships, power struggles in general are predictable. Like those professionals involved in continuing relationships, health care workers have their own way of conducting business. However, as patients and families begin to understand the complexity of their illness and its management, they increasingly take on responsibility for control over their health care.

According to the informants in this study, power struggles were an intensely frustrating element of the health care experience and could occur anytime the patient entered the health care worker's domain. For example, one young man described doing battle with a nurse over having cigarettes in his hospital room:

> I think she was on some sort of a power trip. . . . It got to the point where I got a friend of mine to bring me up a roll of masking tape, and I'd tape my cigarettes to my chest, or my arm. I mean, she'd search everywhere— she'd search the bed (*laugh*). But she'd never search me. . . . She'd leave everything in a total mess, just looking for cigarettes. And she'd take the pillows out of the pillow cases to look for the cigarettes. I mean, it was unbelievable!

An older gentleman recalled a similar power struggle when a nurse insisted that he shave his beard:

> The next day, the same old "battleaxe" come in, and I hadn't shaved for a couple of days, and she started getting into me about not being shaved, and there'd be no beard growing in her ward. . . . When an orderly come with a razor, he was just ready to start shaving me, and I looked at him, and I said, "Lookit, you touch my face with that razor, and you'll be in court on

an assault charge." She was standing right there. She stamped off. . . . I said, "In the first place, I think you better forget all about the war." I says, "You're dealing with the general public now. You haven't got your rank on the shoulder." I says, "I think as far as [this hospital] is concerned, they better put you back emptying bedpans."

From the perspective of these patients and families, power struggles revealed the health care worker's burning need to be right about everything. This attitude further implied that independent decision making on the part of the patient and family was always wrong. For example, Malcolm described an incident in which a doctor seemed to be grasping at straws to find evidence that his independent decision to take his daughter off a therapeutic diet was causing her damage. Although a battery of blood tests did not validate any detrimental effects of the new diet, the doctor insisted that Malcolm's daughter's hair had turned a lighter shade. Thus, from the patient's and the family's point of view, supposedly objective measures were actually manipulated to prove the health care professional's point.

According to many patients and families, rudeness by health care professionals and other workers was a common technique for reinforcing the power imbalance. For example, when one woman asked what she thought was a legitimate question about possible complications for an impending procedure, the doctor "looked at me like I had holes in my head." Another remembered similar rudeness from a nurse when she commented on her daughter's coughing:

I was just so upset, and I still didn't understand what this disease was really. And they tell you things, and it's going right past you, because you can't think, because you're just frozen in time, you're just numb. And I said something to her about the coughing, and she looked at me, and she said, "Well, cystics do cough!" (*abrupt tone of voice*) I was just taken aback, you know, and there was no sympathy, there was nothing, just this cold bitch, that's all she was . . . I don't know how this cold bitch ever got into a kids' hospital.

A third woman recalled an especially rude physician as "standing there like Mr. God in the middle of the room—this arrogant, arrogant ego." According to these patients and families, such rudeness could produce an indelible and unpleasant memory that colored the health care experience considerably.

The struggle for control between the chronically ill and the system was often manifested in the form of a general disrespect for those on the receiving end of health care. As one woman commented, "I find that not often do you find doctors or nurses that want to treat you as somebody who is important, somebody who does know her own body." Many found that their efforts to assert themselves were met with sarcasm or insults. Another manifestation of this disrespect for patients and families involved ridiculing any initiative on their part. One man recalled such an instance:

> When you interviewed me last time I was into my 6th or 7th month of a strange undiagnosed gastric problem that dragged on till only about 4 to 6 weeks ago. And the person who solved it was me! I finally decided I was going to avoid any wheat products, such as pasta or bread. And everything stopped almost overnight! Which leads me to believe that it was a gluten allergy. And I specifically asked my G.P., "Do you think this could be a gluten allergy?" I specifically addressed that question to several specialists and all of them just laughed derisively and said, "Well, if you believe in allergies, then you believe in miracles."

Like many others in this study, this man found that nutrition was an especially popular target for ridicule within the health care system. Interestingly, while most patients and families understood nutrition, stress management, and exercise to be obvious factors in their wellness levels, such attitudes were rarely shared by those with professional credentials.

So for these patients and families, power struggles with health care insiders were unfortunately common—and an inherent outcome of taking on some responsibility for their own health within a system invested in retaining complete control. As one woman explained, this produced a sort of "Catch 22" situation in which acquiescence was the price of access to services. As one woman explained, "That's what brought it to a crisis. . . . People who could help me access what I needed were saying, 'You don't need it because you can tell me what it is. You're just trying to use the system.' " Confrontations over who was in charge were, therefore, an inevitable feature of health care for chronic illness.

Dehumanizing Experiences

A third category of sociocultural confrontation described by the chronically ill individuals and families included encounters that extended the prejudice and power struggle into a context of humiliation and dehumanization. From the perspective of those on the receiving end, the approaches used in this regard were deliberate and cruel. While prejudice and a desire for power were somewhat understandable, these behaviors were not. Thus, the confrontations with the system depicted here represent, from the patient's and family's perspective, a destructive side of humanity incarnate in the health care system.

For patients and families, being treated as if they were children was an intensely humiliating but unfortunately frequent experience. One woman with MS remembered the condescending tone of a young and naive occupational therapist to whom she had confided her serious financial problems:

> She says, "Why don't you go type in the corner?" This was her solution to the whole thing. I mean, years ago I typed, and I ended up typing—I think I was just picking at the thing, 22 words a minute. She said, "That's go-oo-ood." I said, "No, it's no-o-ot. That's not good." One time I tied my shoes and she said, "Oh, that's very good." Patronizing me, you see. . . . You're physically handicapped, but they're trying to make you mentally handicapped.

A man who needed home support services complained of a similarly patronizing attitude from a practical nurse:

> And the last doggone thing when he leaves me, he's got me tucked into bed, and he'll come in and he'll say, "There we are, Mr. J. Bye-bye for now." And he'll pat me on the head. . . . Well, to me, it really is abusive! Because this is patting you on the head like you're a little animal or something.

Being patronized or infantilized represented a source of humiliation for many of these people with chronic illness.

Another form of dehumanization described by the patients and families included remarkable insensitivity to their experience as human beings. For example, one woman recalled going to the surgeon's office to explain in person that her father had died while awaiting his open heart surgery:

> I thought maybe it would look a little nicer than somebody calling and saying, "Sorry, a patient has died." I thought I'd go in and explain to the doctor what happened, and that he wouldn't be coming. The nurse wouldn't let me in to see the doctor. So she said, "Can you leave a message?" I said,

"Yeah, I suppose." And that was hard . . . I had to stand there and say, "Well, there's a patient that was supposed to be coming in here, but he passed away." That was a little bit difficult. I walked out of there not knowing whether I was coming or going. . . . I left my name and informed her, but no, she didn't contact me.

Equally insensitive were some of the conversations between health care workers that patients and families overheard.

I heard one nurse whispering to another, "This is the third one they've brought in tonight." And that innocuous remark, to someone in that sort of crisis, had a horrifying effect on me. I was convinced that this was some sort of a terrible disease. And that's it, these were my last minutes. Look around, this dreary emergency department, and this is it. It's been a slice. Good-bye. Which I think they should teach in medical school and in nursing school—when people are in crisis watch what you say!

Yet another humiliation for many was the way that personal information was considered public knowledge among health care workers. For example, one woman was horrified to see her upcoming appointment for a barium enema advertised on the nursing station chalkboard during visiting hours. Another female patient, a diabetic whose hormones had been fluctuating wildly, recalled her intense embarrassment on being accused of cheating on her diet when it was discovered that her blood sugar was elevated following an outing with a male patient to whom she felt physically attracted.

Invasions of privacy were also described as humiliating and dehumanizing. One woman's account illustrates such an instance:

The day that he told me about the results of the angiogram, we both cried. I had pulled the curtains around his bed, and we both were crying, holding each other's hands. . . . And all of a sudden the curtains whipped open, and—a doctor in a white coat . . . and he said, "Excuse me." And he turned to me again, "Excuse me." So I turned back to [my husband], and it had been obvious we'd both been crying, tears were still there, and I said, "Oh, I'll see you later, honey," whatever, and I walked out. But the way I felt, what I wanted to say to this man (*laugh*), this person in a white coat, was "Who the fuck are you?" It's exactly what I wanted to say to him. I was right in the middle of sharing something with [my husband]. . . . He was invading our privacy.

In addition, a surprising number of patients and family members recounted incidents in which they had been told to "shut up" or "stop crying" by professionals in the health care field. As one young man recalled, "I ended up crying in the bathtub, because there was nobody around."

Other accounts revealed occasions in which withholding information amounted to cruelty from the perspective of the patients and families.

> If I had known on Tuesday that [my son] would be dead by Thursday. . . . Well, shit, I could've sat there, or talked to him, or something. I spent half my time smoking in the lounge, because I didn't know what to do for him (*sobbing*) and it was just so frustrating to sit and look at him. . . . So I said to [the doctor] then, I said, "Look, what is the worst that can happen?" And he wouldn't tell me (*sobbing*). And I came right out and I said to him, "Is he going to die?" And he just said, "I can't answer those questions, you'll have to talk to the surgeon."

Equally cruel were matters of opinion couched as objective facts. One mother of a child with PKU recalled such an instance when she made inquiries about contemplating future pregnancies:

> I mean, I knew the statistics of it. And I said, "What do you think about me having further children? Is it a good idea, or what?" And I can't remember his exact terminology, because he's very, very good at twisting things around, but what he actually in fact said, and how I read it was, "Why would you want to have another child, because if it's another PKU, you're contaminating the world."

Another woman recalled her physician saying to her, "I hate to see what you've cost the system." As she remembered, "I could've fucking decked her right then and there, I was so goddamned mad." Thus, cruel and humiliating interactions were a particularly painful and frustrating type of health care confrontation.

Beyond the insensitivities and cruel encounters that were so bitterly recalled by informants, there were many reports of instances in which these patients and families were treated more as objects than as human beings. One woman recalled such an experience:

> He doesn't drape you, he doesn't cover you up, he doesn't tell you. I mean, you are lying on this old table, which he's probably had for 50 years, with not a stitch on and a sheet over you. He goes through this whole examination. You're on your left side, he's just done a rectal, which is not very comfortable, and then he says, "Turn over," and you get in that goddamned

knee/chest position. And you're not covered up, your whole body is exposed.

According to many of the patients and families, some health care workers seemed incapable of understanding that they were thinking and feeling individuals. As one woman protested, "They're not working on a doll! I could understand that in a doll hospital, you know. My elastic's broken between my arms, you know. But I'm not a doll, and I do know what I feel." The objects of health care rather than its human recipients, these men and women felt painfully dehumanized.

Thus, the social climate of health care was afflicted with a number of attitudes and behaviors perceived as frustrating, humiliating, and even dehumanizing by patients and families. Their experiences in dealing with the human context of health care eventually brought them into contact with profoundly disturbing ideas, policies, and practices. Because they created great anguish, such encounters inevitably shaped an overall opinion about the problems inherent in health care for chronic illness.

CONCLUSIONS

This chapter has drawn from the accounts episode after episode of organizational and sociocultural trauma in the guise of health care for chronic illness. As such, it challenges the reader to acknowledge the dark side of health care as it exists for those enmeshed within it on an ongoing basis. The sheer volume of the anecdotes and the intensity of emotion involved convey a portrait of a system gone wrong. They deny us the possibility of concluding that the problem lies in a particular patient's negativity, the presence of a single "bad apple" in the system, or an unbelievably bad bit of luck. Instead, they are the experiences of real people in a real system, conveyed with the animation and passion that can be discerned in the voices of those who know it best.

The accounts reveal that there are sufficient problems in health care delivery to twist the shape of chronic illness experience beyond recognition. As with the lepers of yesteryear, the physical symptoms of the chronically ill pale in comparison to their social experience in determining what life will be like with disease or disability. The next two chapters will consider in more depth what life with chronic illness becomes when health care fails. They will shift our attention away from the specific miseries within the system and back to the marvelous and miraculous human response that characterizes life for the chronically ill. Thus, they will complete the portrait of chronic illness experience by articulating those dimensions of it that are directly attributable to the experience of being involved in health care in a system such as ours.

EIGHT

Politics and Ideology

Because health care for chronic illness was typically so different from what they had expected and from what they would have thought reasonable, patients and families with chronic illness seemed to devote considerable energy to rationalizing what had gone wrong. For the informants in this study, the process of analyzing the health care system began early in the illness experience and continued with more or less intensity until their ideas had evolved into theories that satisfied their answers to the question, "Why?" On the basis of these interpretations, they could develop increasingly sophisticated strategies for coping with the system's challenges. This chapter will address their interpretations of the system; the next will examine their application of these interpretations to strategic responses.

The ideas patients and families formed addressed their experience in terms of the political structure and ideological foundations of the health care system. In this chapter, a range of theories, showing the ways that various people made sense out of the general difficulties they shared, will be drawn from the accounts. In some cases, the analysis of patients and families was tentative and vague; in others, it was sophisticated and complex. However, underlying all of these theories is the sense that health care and its problems are grounded in the very political and ideological bases of our society. From the various perspectives of the patients and families in this study, the larger picture in health care is one of a system in trouble.

HEALTH CARE POLITICS

Confrontations with the bureaucracy and the logic of health care charged patients and families with reinterpreting the issues of power and control within the system. With each confrontation over time, a new question might be raised and a new answer demanded. Further, the efforts people made to respond to the system fueled additional interpretations. The process of analyzing the system was a prolonged dynamic one, reflecting many variations and diversions over the course of years with chronic illness. The accounts therefore include many interpretations, each drawn from a particular moment in one informant's analytic process.

The politics of health care, according to the informants in this study, included issues having to do with the bureaucratic structure of health delivery, the social structure of professional authority, and the financial structure of health care reimbursement systems. The accounts relating to each of these categories of health care politics reveal the ideas expressed by chronically ill people and their families as to what had gone wrong.

Bureaucratic Structure

Because many of the most frustrating confrontations reflected problems of bureaucracy, many of the patients and families developed ideas about health care organization.

> You know, definitely you experience or see a lot of inadequacies in the health care system, and I think you come to realize that it's not necessarily the people themselves that have caused that—it's just the system as a whole. And I mean, as in any large corporation, or whatever, you're going to run into things that don't run smoothly and need the bugs worked out, you know.

For many, learning the ins and outs of the bureaucratic system was central to understanding their experience. As one woman remarked, "Our system is very labyrinth (*sic*) and you do have to have some knowledge in order to crack the system." Another woman noted that it was a difficult system to learn, "'Cause we're the foreigners there—the aliens."

In analyzing the bureaucratic issues, many patients and families commented on problems inherent in long work hours in demanding roles. As one remarked, "I can appreciate the problem when somebody's there working a 12-hour shift—which I think is bloody ridiculous anyway." In addition, many were aware of staffing shortages and other measures of financial restraint within health care. Like many other patients and families, one woman expressed sympathy for the health care workers caught in a system that deprived them of the opportunity to deliver optimal health care by forcing them to adapt to restraint conditions. "I think a lot of them are overworked and underpaid . . . I think the money is limited, their time is limited, and their caring is." In the view of many, health care funding was either inadequate or improperly directed.

> I've never been like a really political person or activist in anything, but I said, after spending time in the hospital, if I was ever to get up on a soapbox about anything it would be putting more money into the health care system, you know, in whatever way, you know. It could be done with increasing nursing staff, because at 5 o'clock when you see two nurses trying to cope with getting meals to 10 or 12 kids, and the phone's ringing off the hook, and you've got one child up to his ears in poop and another one screaming, and this one tearing around the halls in a wheelchair and knocking everybody else over, you appreciate, you know, what they have to go through. And they need more staff.

Such inadequate funding represented a special worry to the chronically ill who depended on the availability of services, as one man explained:

> They cut the staff, they cut the money, now they're going to go on strike. And I'm sitting here, I have a heart problem and diabetes, and I could go any time. Now, what's going to happen to me if [I get] a heart attack or something and they have no room in the hospital, and I end up in [a nearby town] if I'm lucky. I might be dead by the time I get there.

As has been mentioned, another peculiarity of the bureaucratic health care structure had to do with being required to attend a physician's office in person for such things as test results or prescriptions. When such services did not require any examination, this practice not only created unnecessary waiting but also overloaded the system to the point where interactions between patients and professionals were too hurried. As one man commented, "That's not high-quality care to me. That is revolving-door care." In addition, it defeated attempts at individual responsibility, since access to necessary resources was controlled by these same physicians. One mother protested the contradiction, saying, "It's sort of stupid to go under the assumption that I'm going for their help, because I know what it is she needs."

Further, many commented on faults in the logic of the referral system, which required that these same general practitioners act as gatekeepers for specialists. Although many patients and families understood the general referral principle to be coordination of care, they discovered that actual coordination was almost nonexistent. As one young husband pointed out, the health care system is not really a system in that its parts do not relate to one another. "There doesn't seem to be any concern for the overall care. . . . There's no, like, overall plan. . . . From what we've seen, there is no system there." This lack of overall coordination produced situations such as that of one man who took considerable pains, tying up the system further, to get what he needed:

> I sometimes got referrals from more than one doctor, just because I didn't want to blow my referability. . . . So I had to spread it out a little bit. And be a little bit aware of what type of things. I got certain referrals from certain doctors, and certain ones from other ones.

Similarly, many patients and families commented on the apparent lack of long-term planning within health care in general. From their perspective, relatively minor expenditures toward supportive services could often prevent major costs in acute and long-term care later on. From their perspective, precious resources were wasted because of shortsightedness in health care planning. To many patients and families, the formal health care system seemed far more concerned about diseases than about issues of health and well-being.

> The government doesn't help anybody. All they do, they got their whole priorities screwed up. Most of the system, it's not just the government but most things. Everybody's just doing things on emergency basis—"Oh, that poor kid laying in the gutter, let's pick him up," you know. They don't consider how long it takes to get to the gutter, and the kinds of things that you might do to avoid being in the gutter. . . . And that's probably one of the most frustrating things.

Another somewhat illogical element, according to many of these informants, was the use of physicians as the only legitimate entry point into all other resources within the system. From their point of view, such practices exaggerated the inefficiencies and produced system overload. Thus, according to many chronically ill individuals and their families, the bureaucratic structure of health care explained many of the difficulties they encountered in living with chronic illness. Indeed, some theorized that supporting the infrastructure of the bureaucracy had surpassed even patient care as the priority of the health care system: "Once we turn it into those organizations and those bureaucracies, the philosophy and ideology of those bureaucracies comes to the fore."

For the informants in this study, issues inherent in the health care bureaucracy were to blame for a great deal of the frustration and distress of chronic illness. In fact, one couple claimed that the possibility of contributing to bureaucratic change was their primary reason for volunteering to be interviewed for this study:

> We've come to terms, and we know what we have to do, and stuff, and it's easier now because we just do what we have to do. But for the people that are coming, you know—the people in the future—what are they going to have? Are they going to go through the same crap that we've had to go through, too? How many lives are going to be wrecked? . . . It's stupid!

From their point of view, if the people in charge truly appreciated the issues, they would surely be motivated to correct the bureaucratic nightmares that make chronic illness so frustrating.

Professional Authority

A second aspect of health care politics analyzed by the patients and families in this study involved relationships among and between health care professionals of various persuasions. As they increased their contact with the system, people began to develop theories about the way the professions socialized their members and the way each understood its unique contribution to health care. They also began to recognize how professional behaviors and territorial battles influenced the conduct of health care within the system.

According to many patients and families, physicians with caring attitudes were a rare breed. As one woman remarked, "I'm sure there are some doctors out there that really do give a damn. . . . I think they're in the minority, but I know there are some out there." Interestingly, this woman was among those patients who had a physician within the immediate family. A common observation was that physicians seemed unprepared to deal with the emotional component of health problems:

> I think a lot of GPs, or physicians, and/or specialists, whatever, can cope with the physical stuff, but they cannot cope with the emotional. It's almost as though you need a psychiatrist when things are real rough, and deal with the emotions.

In the opinion of many patients and families, this characteristic aversion to emotional expression could be attributed to medical education. As one patient concluded, "I guess he's just not trained in things in the brain and in the emotions. He's a physician and he deals with broken bones and colds and that kind of thing."

Another professional characteristic noted by many was a disinclination to be honest with patients. Because being honest with people about their chronic illness could provoke intense emotional responses, many patients and families thought physicians withheld information in order to protect themselves. One woman explained why she found this attribute unforgivable:

> Subconsciously, we knew that things were pretty serious here, but he wasn't about to bring them on to a conscious level and come right out with it. And I found it was almost an insult to us, you know, like we were intelligent people, we had been dealing with this for a long time, we were prepared. We need to prepare for the bottom line, you know. And I think that's an area that doctors have trouble dealing with.

In contrast, others surmised that the lack of honesty they experienced was more generally attributable to the typical physician's aversion to admitting that he or she did not have all the answers. Thus, many patients and families described the professional character of physicians as uncaring, withholding, and uncomfortable with the emotional dimensions of chronic illness.

The informants also described a character they typically associated with nurses, the other major health care professional group with whom most had some degree of personal experience. According to many patients and families, the typical nurse was generally quite accessible and accepting.

> The nurses that I've met, and that I've talked to, are more apt to treat me equally, and to talk to me—like to share with me what knowledge they've got about what I'm going through. They don't seem to want to lay trips on me, or be the professional with all the answers, who's going to prescribe something that is going to magically make it all better for me.

For many, this accessibility included being willing to take time with patients and families and to engage in "nonprofessional" conversation. In contrast, however, some patients and families found that informal interaction could also be frustrating. "I really don't like when the nurses come in and gossip about other patients." Further, many informants noted major discrepancies between what they considered good nurses and poor nurses:

> There are certain nurses over the course of the various hospitalizations that have been exceptional, you know—not only competent, but have been extremely caring, and those we have honored. There are other nurses that really don't bring honor to themselves or their profession—by their laziness and incompetence, and their whole demeanor.

In addition, they noted marked differences in the behavior of nurses in different settings. Their ideas about the behavior of nurses clearly indicated that, from the perspective of chronically ill individuals and families, human interaction is an important attribute of good nursing.

For many informants, the characteristics of the two professions were symbolized by the contrasting behaviors between doctors and nurses. Their accounts of these distinctions revealed various explanations. According to some patients and families, doctors had less time than did nurses. "I guess with the doctor, maybe there's a little more the sense that he's really busy so you don't bother him. You deal—like the system is, you deal through the nurse." Further, they were seen as more distant from the people for whom they were caring. "The nurses are the ones that are there doing it all the time. The doctors are very remote."

According to many patients and families, a social status differential set physicians apart from their patients more than it did nurses:

> I think it's not so much that you have more respect for doctors than nurses, but just the fact that you can sort of feel that with the nurse she's more on your level, you know. You can tell dirty jokes, or whatever, you know. Whereas the doctor, they're sort of that one step above, you know, it's not quite the same . . . there's still always that fine line there.

From their perspective, the inherent social distance between patients and physicians was maintained by the behavior of both parties. As one man explained, "Doctors, sometimes, they may think they're communicating, but they aren't. They either use those big words or they're in such a rush they don't have time to talk." Further, many suspected that the relative positions of the nurses and doctors within the health care hierarchy influenced the way patients and families reacted to them.

> Maybe it's because the nurses that I've seen are not really in charge of the reason why I'm going in, like the nurse is there to assist the doctor. The doctor's the one I'm asking the answers from. And I mean, I might not get the answers from a doctor, that would leave me with doubts about the doctor, but not necessarily about the nurse. . . . You can't really be upset with the nurse for following orders. I would not yell at a waitress for bringing me something that the cook burned.

From their vantage point, then, the distinctions between nurses and doctors were significant factors in understanding some of the conflict within health care.

Appreciating the characteristic social qualities of various health care professions also helped patients and families make sense of the intense conflict they began to observe between factions within the formal and informal health care system. Because many chronically ill people had considered alternatives to traditional medical practice at some point in their illness experience, they had noticed intense friction between the diverse health care orientations. According to these patients and families, territorial battles between the medical profession and all other health care orientations were especially frustrating.

> For instance, doctors will not give you a recommendation to a chiropractor. They'll say to go to a physiotherapist. . . . And then we start getting into all the politics of the medical profession. And, quite frankly, when I'm in pain, I don't give a damn about the politics. Just tell me what I can do, where I can go, that will help me, you know. And when I start seeing those roadblocks, that's frustrating.

From their perspective, this conflict was fueled by the medical profession's conviction that its orientation to health issues was exclusively valid. Since curative treatment was unlikely in the event of chronic disease, physicians were often defensive about their authority in chronic illness care, as one man's comments illustrate:

> The more defensive a physician feels, the more arrogant he or she is, because they are trying to compensate for their insecurity. And medicine now is under attack, so they are much more defensive and much more arrogant in its behavior to patients.

Beyond identifying territorial wars between practitioners of various orientations, chronically ill people and their families were aware of battles for control within the medical care system itself. Again, they often remarked on medicine's struggle for authority over the other health professions, especially nurses.

> I've also known enough nurses to realize who does most of the real caregiving. I've seen enough situations where nurses are really in charge and doctors are de facto in charge and get a lot of the limelight for it. I have a lot more confidence in the caregiving that nurses dispense because I think nurses are closer to patients. They feel a greater responsibility.

Another patient theorized that differences in education between doctors and nurses are exaggerated in the formal system of authority. "He studies for 2 more years than the nurse, but does that mean he's God?" While the majority of such conflict was observed between nurses and physicians, several patients and families observed that it carried on down through the ranks, so that worth was measured more by professional status than by expertise.

While much of the political turmoil observed in health care occurred between the various professions and orientations to medicine, many informants also noticed political overtones in the relationships between members of the same profession. According to these people, the tangibly different morale levels on various hospital units were a product of relations between the head nurse and his or her staff. Another political issue of concern to many chronically ill people and families was the "old-boys' network" they perceived among members of the medical profession. In their opinion, the spirit of medical fraternity often blinded physicians to the failings of their colleagues. Further, many patients and families were distressed by an unwritten understanding among physicians that prevented their attending to aspects of the patient that were within a colleague's domain. According to many informants, this territorial understanding among physicians was probably financially motivated.

> I think it's very much protecting your own territory. I think it's also a certain amount of politics and obviously, where politics is involved, money is involved. . . . There's all kinds of politics in the medical profession [that] I think prevents a level of patient care from occurring. I don't think any of the people would admit that.

Thus, the men and women living with chronic illness articulated problems in the politics of professional authority as explanations of some of their difficulties in obtaining appropriate health care. From their point of view, the professions were distinct from each other by virtue of certain identifiable characteristic types of behavior and the hierarchical structure within health care. However, from their perspective, the hierarchy often interfered with their ability to obtain the care they needed, and certainly produced considerable conflict within the system. As their experience in the system evolved, many of these people came to interpret such conflict as a struggle for power rather than a concern about competence.

Financial Incentives

From the perspective of chronically ill patients and their families, the financial interests of those involved in the health care industry explained a great deal about why the system functioned in the way it did. As Canadian residents, the informants in this study were all entitled to insured health care, for which they were universally grateful. In particular, many compared their situation to that of their American cousins. As a mother of two asthmatic children explained:

> I'm really grateful that we're up here, where they have a medical system that takes care of little kids that are sick. 'Cause we'd probably owe them $50,000 if we were paying them for every time they had a croup attack.

However, many of the patients and families in this study had gone beyond what was insured in their search for health care. From their point of view, it was worth paying these expenditures out of pocket if they made a difference to their well-being. Thus, while they were grateful for the insured system, many paid for additional health care when the system did not meet their needs.

As earlier discussions revealed, many patients and families expressed concern about the way the medical services remuneration system influenced decisions about their health care. For example, they recognized that it encouraged doctors to insist on office visits, for which they could be reimbursed, rather than brief telephone consultations. From their perspective, this remuneration system linked doctors' salaries to their efficiency.

> I don't know if this is true, but I have a sense that doctors have some kind of an unspoken quota in their head about how many patients they have to

go through to make a certain amount of money. . . . I don't know how
doctors determine that, how many appointments they book or whatever.
There must be some kind of a system.

Many patients and families believed that doctors tended to increase
the size of their practices to a point at which optimal care was impossible. As one patient complained, "He's not interested in his patient. He
is interested in the bucks that he's going to get out of what he's doing."
Further, many thought that the pressures of remuneration influenced the
personal attention that was possible, even from the most caring of
practitioners. As one patient complained, "You seem to get one guy
who's nice like that and cares, and word gets out. And before you know
it, he's got a huge clientele, and then he becomes very busy and he has
a hard time dealing with so many patients."

Patients often described the climate of doctor's offices by using such
phrases as "going through a revolving door" or "being cranked through
the mill." In their perception, patient overload and the resultant lack of
personalized care were understood to be a by-product of the remuneration system. Another presumed effect of remuneration's influence on
medical decisions was reflected in the belief that doctors' salaries were
dependent on the number of patients they hospitalized. For example,
one woman linked a doctor's unwillingness to discharge her husband
from hospital to the possibility that it might reduce his reimbursement
from the medical plan. Many patients also suspected that remuneration
policies played a role in the reluctance of some practitioners to advocate
home care or outpatient services.

Referrals were also believed to be influenced by financial implications. As one woman wondered, "Well, are doctors afraid to refer to a
specialist? Is there some sort of financial loss or some status loss if they
do refer you?" In contrast, others suspected that physicians had financial arrangements with one another, as well as with various laboratories
and hospitals, to provide a cut of the profits in exchange for referrals:
"Sometimes he sends me there because he probably gets a cut in the
rate." Thus, patients and families came to suspect that reimbursement
policies unduly influenced professional clinical decisions.

Another observation made by the informants in this study was that
the health insurance scheme created a climate in which overconsump-
tion was rampant. While many recognized that some patients might
abuse the services, others found health care professionals to be equally
wasteful. For example, patients noted the overuse of lab testing for no

diagnostic or treatment benefit, and an excess of prescription medications, as evidence of a socially irresponsible attitude toward consumption within the health care system.

> I think that we've been brought up to be very wasteful. And so that goes as well for the health care system. I just think that a lot of prescriptions are made that don't necessarily need to be made. I think we're acting very weird.

Further, many chronically ill individuals and families thought that the universality of health insurance had made health professionals quite unconcerned about the actual costs involved in their decisions.

> They tried a new drug, and the prescription cost us $526. . . . I phoned [the doctor], and I said, "Do you realize, Doctor, that the prescription is $526?" And he says, "You know you're getting it back from the government. You've got the money." Well, I mean, we could pay for it, but it's just the principle.

Many patients and families came to realize, through the course of their illness experience, that their continued involvement in health care ensured the continuing salary of their physicians. Thus, many came to suspect that specialists in chronic illness might be in the business not for reasons of altruism or science, but for the purpose of generating a sizable income. As one woman explained:

> When it comes to MS . . . I think they found the most cushy deal. I really do. . . . Now, if I was a doctor I would think, "I am going to have my complete patient load be MS people. All I have to do is smile, send them off to a shrink, or the MS Society, or the support group."

So the idea that their continuing illness represented the livelihood of their professional health care providers was an unsettling thought for many.

In a similar vein, many chronically ill patients and families developed an awareness of the degree to which their illnesses represented a potential profit for other members of the health care industry. Medical conferences were often mentioned as a means of generating profits. Those who had attended several expressed dismay at the lack of scholarly enthusiasm by the professionals attending, and at the fees patients had been charged in order to attend. "They're not even looking [to help] somebody who's got damage. . . . I think it all has to do with meetings, and how to make a fortune on those crummy lunches." A related profit potential noted by many informants was the direct relationship between the medical profession and the pharmaceutical industry. Some thought that the industry had altered medical practice beyond recognition: "I now am a bit, as you can probably tell, a bit cynical about the traditional medical approach. . . . I now know that they're primarily, to me, dispensers of medicine." Clearly, the frequency with which medical conferences were sponsored by pharmaceutical corporations further raised suspicions that there were profits to be made from their ongoing illness.

One aspect of health care economics that greatly concerned many patients and families in this study was priorities in research funding. Because many thought research to be a source of hope for their future, they were most distressed to discover that its funding, too, was political. For example, many considered the overall expenditure on health care research insignificant in comparison to other areas of public funding. Like others, one woman was quite convinced that failures in medical research were more directly linked to funding priorities than they were to the limitations of science:

> This is the most aggravating thing, knowing that the treatment can be found. . . . You can't tell me 40 years from when they first found out about the white blood cells being very responsible for it. . . . You've got to go through a world war, and [a man on] the moon, and you can't tell me they couldn't have found some treatment, some better treatment for not only MS, but a lot of the diseases, you know, Cystic Fibrosis. I feel, you know, that the priorities are all wrong.

Further, many found that health care research was concentrated in a few highly publicized fields, to the exclusion of many types of chronic illness: "Like Lupus is getting quite a bit of money now for research because they've gained national recognition." As one woman with Scleroderma explained, patients need to become involved in creating a public profile before they could hope for adequate research support. However, in spite of their own willingness to fund-raise and become involved, many informants recognized that the interest of medical researchers was critical to the success of any research program. To their dismay, they discovered that competition between such researchers for prestige and recognition may have inhibited scientific progress.

> Oh, the United States and Canada decided to share their information, their findings in research. Do you find anything stupid about that? That they've

been spending millions here, and across the border a few miles away they've been spending millions on the same research and they haven't been sharing. They're very egotistical, right? Mr. So-and-so wants to be the one who comes up with this. While all these people are sitting around in wheelchairs, they're fighting over who gets the credit in the *New England Journal of Medicine*!

Thus, the economic potential of chronic illness made many patients and families highly attuned to how funds were used and who stood to profit from them.

A final concern with regard to the economics of health care was raised by many chronically ill individuals and families in the course of the study. Although aware that their theories might be considered paranoid by others, many expressed the opinion that there might be a better financial incentive in keeping them ill than in providing them with either curative or supportive services. As they surveyed the economic landscape, several informants noticed that the health care bureaucracy was in fact a complex industry whose basic market depended upon maintaining a certain level of illness in society.

We build monuments and have created an industry to cancer, while in turn, a very large numbers of the cancers that there are, we create. So we have a nice dialectic in that we have technology that creates machines, and medication to deal with the cancers, which we create with all these carcinogenic substances that we have, and out of those too we fund research to look into creating ways to deal with creating new fertilizers, or new substances that are noncarcinogenic, and also to create new substances that deal with how we cure cancer. But it's an industry that—each part of the fundamental industry, where there is the hospital, the pharmaceuticals, the engineering, whatever—feeds upon each other. They need each other in order to continue to survive, so they have no real vested interests in finding a cure.

From their various perspectives, many patients and families came to question the effect of financial incentives on this very basic premise of health care. As one woman remarked, "That's one thing in the back of your mind . . . they don't want us to be cured because it's, you know, their bread and butter." From their perspective, health care professionals might be unwitting parties to the shift toward this new objective.

I don't quite know how to explain it, but it almost seems as though the health care system is set up, and people are brought to a certain level of health, and then there's a sort of, "Well, we can't make everybody healthier, we'll be phased out of our jobs, and there goes our work" (*laugh*)—So that you're consistently a consumer of that system. And I'm sure that that's not a conscious plot, I think that that's just the way it's happened.

As a result, with increasing horror and dismay, many chronically ill individuals and their families toyed with the idea that the health care system itself might have an investment in their misery.

The accounts therefore reflected considerable concern about the extent to which financial interests influence health care politics. One man's conclusion revealed a deep distrust for the profit potential that had twisted the shape of medical care during his lifetime:

The way the medical field has evolved . . . there's no doubt about it that it's a very mercenary thing by a lot of them. It's a business. . . . In the field of anything where we are dollar motivated, the better qualities of human beings are subverted. . . . The whole objective is to make money.

For this man and for many others, the role of economics in explaining some of the frightening problems in health care delivery was inescapable.

The accounts presented here illustrate the extent to which chronically ill people and their families understand health care politics to be a source of many of their serious confrontations with health care. Although their interpretations represent various degrees of sophistication and analysis, they consistently reveal that those involved with chronic illness experience power and money as influential factors in their lives. They identify the tendency of a bureaucracy to sustain itself, the tendency of professional bodies to promote themselves, and the tendency of industry to seek profit as social forces having a direct bearing on their quality of life with chronic illness. Therefore, they encourage us to recognize that chronic illness experience must be interpreted in the context of health care politics to be understood.

HEALTH CARE IDEOLOGY

The second focus of analysis articulated by patients and their families in their efforts to understand their experiences in health care reflected the assumptions and beliefs that underpin the structure and function of the health care system. As was noted earlier, the informants in this study described themselves as entering the chronic illness experience with a rather blind faith in the system's benevolence and in its ability to resolve health problems. Because this faith was inevitably challenged, people had occasion to wonder about its origins and develop theories about how our culture constructs its ideas about health care. Thus, they interpreted many of their experiences in terms of what they came to understand as health care ideology.

The patients and their families articulated three distinct components of what they considered a widespread belief system about health care. The first of these was that doctors know what is best for patients; the second was that "regular" medicine is superior to all other healing practices; and the third was that medicine was a precise form of scientific enterprise. Their accounts illustrate how they came to challenge each of these beliefs.

The Doctor Knows Best

The informants all admitted to entering the chronic illness experience with an attitude of reverence toward doctors. For example, one woman remembered herself as "really believing in God the Almighty Doctor." Another explained a similar awe:

> I used to think of a hospital, or doctors, as more or less like mini-gods, you know, if you were sick you put yourself in this guy's care, and he took care of you, and that was it, you know. You never questioned whether it was good or bad, or what.

A third noted that a physician's "word was gospel" on any topic related or unrelated to health care. However, invariably, chronic illness shook the foundations of this belief. As they learned to appreciate their own expertise in this regard, the informants also began to understand the role their beliefs had played in causing them to look to professionals for answers they could not provide. The experience of chronic illness brought patients and their families to the realization that doctors do not know everything, and that, in particular, they may know very little about what constitutes everyday life with chronic illness.

In shifting their own attitudes, patients and families began to recognize that their views were consistent with those of others in similar circumstances. Further, they identified common patterns in the way people rely upon their doctors. They recognized that there were cases in which professionals were incapable of providing help because the patients were overly dependent.

> I think for health professionals, one of the hardest things must be getting people with attitudes that they just don't care and they're not going to try. . . . What I have heard people say who work in the health profession is, they find it difficult to work with people like alcoholics or heroin addicts, just 'cause they keep doing it over and over again.

However, they also noted that many patients simply were not aware of any alternative to seeking help from physicians when they had physical symptoms.

> I understand that doctors are subjected to requests from patients who would be better off being treated in some other way. But they don't know any other way, and that's why they go to these doctors. That's why they continue to go to the doctor even though the illness may be treated in some other way—it could be dealt with at home or, given a little time, will resolve itself. But they don't know that.

In addition, some appreciated that going to the doctor had additional cultural meanings for some patients. As one man theorized, "I think a lot of people go to MDs for reassurance as much as they go for medicine or actual help." In conjunction with depending too much on doctors, many informants commented on the tendency of people to avoid taking personal responsibility for their health.

> We can't expect by leading a sort of unhealthy life, which we do to a certain extent, to be cured and in good health, you know. We can't expect the physicians to cure us for something he has no foundation for, you know, because we don't make the foundation.

By shifting their own interpretation away from the ideology of "doctor knows best," many patients and families found themselves more accepting of the limitations of their own physicians.

The other side of the argument with regard to unrealistic expectations, however, was the role physicians played in cultivating an impression of their omnipotence. In spite of the physicians' inability to offer meaningful services in chronic illness, many informants claimed that they considered themselves infallible healers. "I kind of think that the medical profession tends to cater to that, too, with prescriptions, and with just quick fixes." From their perspective, this inflated self-image was the reason that physicians expected to have a monopoly on services for the chronically ill. "Society has given these people the role of expert. And you go there, and they don't have answers, or they have answers that don't make any sense to you, because they're not of your reality." However, from their standpoint such an attitude was completely inappropriate in the context of many chronic illnesses. "In an area where there are no real answers anyway, they seem to think that they have the right to dictate in a very unfeeling way to you, what you should do, and what you should not do." Thus, many believed that the attitudes of doctors played a role in producing the unrealistic expectations of their clients.

Another way in which doctors were perceived as contributing to the problem was in their unwillingness to consider their patients credible. As one man explained, "I think some of them say, 'Well, I'm the doctor, you're the patient.' And that's an attitude I heard from many people." Many of these patients and families expressed some sympathy for the physicians in this regard, since they surmised that it must be frustrating to be challenged by patients. "I think it's really frustrating for the doctors, because they feel like, I've gone to school for 10 years, and I've practiced, and this guy is going to question my diagnostic procedures." Further, they understood that chronic illness must pose an especially embarrassing challenge to those trained for the purpose of treatment and cure. "I'm sure it bothers them to know that there's not a damn thing they can do overall." Thus, for many patients and families, much of the conflict in health care for chronic illness could be understood in terms of the unrealistic expectation held by both the general public and the medical profession that the doctor was the only legitimate expert in matters having to do with health. One patient's recollections reveal her realization that the power of the doctor in all such affairs was a sham:

> It was that sort of experience . . . that makes people particularly bitter and disillusioned with the god. And the god that failed. Some people are great believers in the ideology and realize that ideology was a failure. Well, in my case I guess the ideology was that physical medicine can help. . . . And you gradually realize that it's not so.

The Superiority of Regular Medicine

Although some of the patients and families in this study had been exposed to nontraditional healing arts, home remedies, and alternative therapies prior to their diagnosis with chronic illness, none began their health care experience with any doubt that regular medicine was superior. For many, this belief was a profound article of faith. As one patient explained, "I always believed it was only the medical profession, technical professionals, could treat illness. I mean, it was their purview, their sanctuary."

The depth of this belief was illustrated in the accounts of patients and families considering alternatives in the early stages of their illness. One woman recalled needing symbolic legitimacy from someone aligned with traditional medicine before she could consider the credibility of an alternative:

> I guess I heard about [the naturopath], it would've been a year, or 2 years before. And it was through a lady in our church, who is an RN, who got into this area of holistic medicine, and naturopathy . . . and she was very much against going to a chiropractor or anything . . . just going through medical. And so when she got interested in it, I mean, she really researched it. So it was like when she told me about it, it was like, "Well, I can accept this," because here's an RN who knows the medical side, and she's saying this other has validity. . . . I was really skeptical.

Similarly, a male patient recalled his initial cynicism: "Anything that wasn't logic, I didn't want anything to do with that, you know. I didn't want anybody dancing around me, and sprinkling herbs on me." From his perspective, such skepticism was a natural outcome of widespread "negative press about alternative health care." As another patient concluded, "It takes a lot to desocialize that emphasis on traditional health care."

In spite of this skepticism, many of the patients and families in this study did eventually pursue a course not prescribed by their regular doctors. In some cases, they simply altered their diets, took vitamins or health food supplements. In other instances, they engaged in prolonged therapies under the guidance of acupuncturists, naturopaths, homeopaths, chiropractors, native healers, or psychics. Such adventures into alternative therapies were often driven by desperation.

> If you're not getting helped, then you're going to go somewhere else. You'll say, okay, what else can I investigate? And I think it's at that point of frustration that you reach in not getting help, and this sends people to the Philippines so some guy can pull pieces of cow intestine out of them. I mean, it's whatever it takes.

More often, however, they were fueled by a growing sense that important aspects of their complex situations were not considered in the traditional medical approach. As they began to recognize the extent to which their psyches influenced their symptoms, and their nutrition influenced their energy levels, for example, these patients and families sought alternative approaches that they thought capable of appreciating illness in a more holistic framework.

As many pointed out, their own skepticism did not really disappear until an alternative treatment actually worked:

> I thought [applied kinesiology] was off the wall myself. It is strange when you try and describe it to somebody. You say, hold your fingers in certain positions and they flick your ears, and people look at you as if you just climbed off the spaceship! So it was quite bizarre, and I had to overcome a certain amount of cynicism that I had. But I wouldn't have overcome any of that if it hadn't worked.

Once they had obtained symptom relief or other benefits from an alternative, however, they were convinced. One mother, for example, was delighted at the success of chiropractic in treating her son with CP. "I don't care what a lot of people say if they're against chiropractors. Since we've been taking [my son] to him, he's holding his head up, and I'm not going to take that away from him." Similarly, a young man described his success in reducing chronic back pain through the guidance of a naturopath:

> It was, "What are the triggers for this? What is making this pain happen here?" That impressed me! I mean, I'm a logical person, and that's the first time that I thought that somebody was approaching my back pain in a logical way. . . . And I find that ironic, I guess . . . because I put a lot of credence in the medical profession, and it hadn't delivered, and I put so little credence in something I was quite skeptical about, and then had it deliver.

Success with alternative treatments caused many patients and families to contrast the theories underlying them with those inherent in traditional medicine. One woman, for example, pointed to the frequency with which medicine ignores abuse as an underlying source of human distress. A young man theorized that many physical symptoms could be attributed to such social factors: "It's a warning system, I guess. Not letting your energies flow the way they should flow." Many pointed out that the notion of energy circulation, basic to Eastern healing practices, was completely overlooked in Western medicine: "I think those people have a lot to share with us of the Western world." Others noted that medicine had not kept pace with environmental changes in determining such issues as nutrition:

> Our soil has been depleted and our soil is being poisoned with the fallout from car emissions . . . so your soil is not like what it used to be years ago. So you have to take supplements to get your vitamins and minerals.

Although they became enthusiastic about alternative health promotion and treatment methods, most patients and families saw themselves as informed and rational consumers rather than desperate cure-seekers. They therefore made clear distinctions between what they considered quackery and legitimate approaches:

> Somebody gave me a book about distilled water. Incredibly poorly written, and I can't imagine how people would be taken in. . . . I sometimes have a big laugh (*laugh*) because you can see right through some of those things . . . I just got a book in the mail and it was another one of those Biblical ones—You can cure yourself if you believe this. That one really worries me more than any others.

Thus, their experiences in alternative methods were a source of comfort and relief for many patients, and a challenge to their earlier faith in the superiority of medicine. For most, each system of understanding health problems had its strengths and limitations. In this way, many of the patients and families found themselves asking penetrating questions about the superiority of the biomedical approach to health.

In conjunction with their own growing acceptance of alternative philosophies of health and healing, chronically ill individuals and their families were increasingly concerned about the basis for the resistance most medical practitioners held toward such approaches. In addition, they began to appreciate that medical logic was incapable of dealing with issues of human variation sufficiently to allow for the possibility that individual benefits might be distinct from those that could be proven as generalizations. As one woman explained, while doctors saw diseases as single entities, patients were more likely to understand that each individual's chronic illness was different: "I'm not sure that there's anybody else out there that's got exactly the same kind of asthma I've got, you know, any more than we look alike (*laugh*) sort of thing." From their point of view, this was a serious flaw in medical thinking.

> They only look at the technical, the clinical side of it . . . they're not looking at the other side of it: How does my body react as a whole person? And therefore I lose that sense of trust in them.

Their own generally positive experiences, combined with their physicians' generally negative attitudes about the alternatives, created serious doubt about the superiority of regular medicine in managing chronic illness. From the perspective of these patients and families, the medical profession was missing important clues because of its narrow approach to interpreting health problems:

> I find it really ironic that at [the arthritis center] there's a lot of older crippled people sitting around, and a cart comes through, with a volunteer pushing the most awful packaged chemically loaded cookies, coffee out of an old tin, a big bowl of sugar, you know, and that's what they're feeding them. So, you know, I believe in a balanced sort of traditional and nontraditional type medicine. And I do believe that there is a place for very traditional medicine, drugs and all that, but I think that there's a lot of room for the other also. And I think probably a lot of people do things on their own, and they just never tell the doctor.

The Logic of Medical Science

Recognizing that their physicians were not merely being impolite but rather were voicing the objections inherent in their approach to illness, many chronically ill people and families eventually began to rethink the objectivity and precision of medical science itself. Some came to the conclusion that what appeared to be scientific precision was merely the law of averages. An asthmatic woman made the following observations about drug therapy:

> You can't find a doctor that will ever tell you one puff. They all say two puffs of Ventolin. Now I get along really well many, many days with one puff. Why would I take two? If I can control this on one puff, I don't see any reason why I need to take two.

And a diabetic man had similar concerns about controlled diets:

It doesn't matter what you do, you know. If you're at home laying in bed, she will give you the same diet, according to the weight. If I'm 200 pounds laying in bed, she will give me that diet. If I'm 200 pounds working like a dog in lumber, she will give me the same diet. Know what I mean? It's not gonna work the same.

In both of these instances, the patients believed that the imprecision of the treatment order was beyond the comprehension of their physician. One woman explained why she thought this was so: "The system in and of itself . . . does not look at the individual per se. It tends to look at the disease."

Some patients and families also began to recognize that medical science was often simply a matter of guesswork. One mother, for example, was astounded at the rather simplistic logic applied to definitive diagnosis: "I think it's kinda strange that the only real definition of having asthma is that, if these asthma medications improve your condition, you've got it. . . . Weird, eh?" Further, many began to understand that the guesswork was based only upon highly selective information. For example, one man's elementary observations link factors that he thought were generally ignored in the "scientific" approach to understanding illness:

I don't know if you noticed, but poverty brings infirms in family. There's so many infirms—children with only one eye, you know, and children all crippled up . . . In Mexico, and the small towns in Quebec, I saw the same thing. A lot of people have infirms in their family. And I really have to question. Poverty and infirms come together, it seems to me.

And another patient observed, "We label too many people hypochondriacs, but they die often within 5 years. And hypochondria shouldn't kill anybody!"

Their awareness of these peculiarities in medical thinking led many patients and families to the conclusion that much of the knowledge derived from medical science was a matter of opinion rather than truth. As one young man noted, "You come out with stats about this works better, this works better with this type of person—but it's still opinionated." Further, they also developed the realization that a science in progress was always an idea pending refutation:

Medical science has a long way to go, and they don't have the answer for everything, and what was true yesterday is not true today. The treatment of yesterday has been discarded, and a new treatment is given today. So you know . . . science marches on.

Thus, their sense of the relationship between facts and science caused them to further doubt the absolute applicability of medical science to human problems.

In addition, some patients and families commented on other issues in which the supposed objectivity of medicine was debatable. One woman, for example, discovered that the concept of a "rare disease" actually referred more to the extent of medical knowledge about it than it did to statistical indicators of prevalence:

> When they're taught about Scleroderma in medical school . . . they learn that Scleroderma's a rare disease. They learn that there is no cure for it. . . . There's no in-depth education, so the doctor doesn't know what to look for . . . because it's still the mentality that is there, that this is so rare.

Another discovered that disease names were merely indicators of categories of human problems that medicine assumed shared some similarity:

> I think we're dealing with a lot of different diseases here, and they've grouped it all together as MS. . . . I think it's a lot of other diseases, and it's like one of those things where, at the end of the day, and there's a bunch of junk here and you just swoop it all into one drawer, you know?

Such insights shocked many chronically ill individuals and families into a profound questioning of the rationality of medical science. As one woman explained, she had never previously considered the possibility that medical science "was incapable of a very thorough, rational approach to my problems." In many cases, such insight led to doubts about medical research. As one woman came to believe, such research served to foster an unreal optimism about cure while diverting resources from the very real living problems of patients:

> There is nothing constructive . . . I don't see anything in the future but more of this MS research bullshit. There's no hope of ever getting a job. There's no hope of me being an independent person, there's no hope. And I will end up on Welfare again . . . still receiving two letters a year from the MS Society, telling me about their research.

So many came to an understanding of medical science as simply a system of beliefs, rather than a window into the truth.

In considering the beliefs inherent in medical science, some of the men and women in this study came to rather chilling conclusions. For example, many began to see medical science as the organ of a death-denying culture. From their perspective, the failings of medical science reflected much larger ideological problems in society, including the failure to examine the long-range impact of major social decisions. As one woman commented:

> To me, Prednisone is like the atomic bomb of the internal cellular level of the being. . . . And it horrifies me that some physicians seem to be rolling these drugs out as a kind of first or second defense system, instead of as an absolutely last possible alternative.

Like others for whom chronic illness had brought new ways of understanding the world, this woman believed that the dark side of medical progress was barely recognized by society at large.

Thus, their chronic illness experience brought many patients and families to a new appreciation for the ideology underlying medical science. As one man explained:

> I think that we've been sold a bill of goods, and we've swallowed the notion that there is a small number of people who go to school and learn a certain thing and that's called medicine. And we come to expect that they can intervene and solve problems which we consider to be medical problems. And to an extent I think that's a consequence of the medical profession gaining a monopoly on the delivery of health services. . . . But we originally start out believing . . . from a nonreligious, nonmystical, very science-oriented background . . . that there is something called medical science.

By rethinking the bases of their belief that the doctor knows what is best for people, that regular medicine is superior to all other healing approaches, and that medical science is the key to the questions of health and illness, the patients and families in this study challenged the very ideological foundations of the health care system. With varying sophistication, in relation to different issues, and from a range of perspectives, many came to the conclusion that health care, the way it is currently conducted, is a matter of deeply embedded belief systems.

CONCLUSIONS

Chronically ill people analyze the health care system in order to make sense of what has happened to them within it. According to the informants in this study, many of the experiences encountered by the chronically ill in the health care system can be explained in the context of health care politics and health care ideology. From their perspective, the health care bureaucracy has become so complex that its primary incentive is to sustain itself rather than to organize the delivery of health care to sick people. Because of its peculiarities in regulations and policies, the health care bureaucracy creates a major source of frustration for chronically ill patients and families.

Another source of frustration for these people is the territorial conflicts between the various stakeholders in health care. Their experiences over time allow them to witness considerable conflict between professions, between schools of thought, and between individual practitioners. In addition, patients and families begin to understand the financial investment that the health care industry represents in our society. From their perspective, profit motives explain many aspects of policy, procedure, and even professional decision making. Further, many of those afflicted by chronic illness also start to appreciate the degree to which they represent a lucrative natural resource for the health care industry.

The second component of the analysis is the ideology that supports the political structure of health care. Because their experiences demand that they reevaluate their own ideas about health, illness, and conditions for wellness, those living with chronic illness begin to understand health care as founded upon a set of shared beliefs, assumptions, and values. They are forced to rethink their own socialized dependence upon physicians as the sole authority on matters of the body. In so doing, they begin to recognize the existence of competing worldviews, some trendy and others as old as time, that may provide the key to an enhanced quality of life with chronic illness. Because their successes in this regard are met with derision and resistance by most medical practitioners, the chronically ill and their families begin to question the very foundations of medical science. While few could articulate a formal defense of their analysis, and few could construct a scholarly criticism of scientific principles, there is ample evidence for those who choose to look that these chronically ill people gradually develop a critical outlook upon the major questions of ideology within science.

The accounts have demonstrated the extent and depth of analysis required by the chronically ill to make sense of their experience in health care. By coming to understand the larger context of their distress, people with chronic illness and their families form an analytic basis on which to refine their coping strategies and thereby navigate the troubled waters of health care more smoothly and certainly.

NINE

Response and Resolution

In this chapter, we will consider the accounts of how chronically ill individuals and families respond to the problems in the health care system and resolve, to the best of their ability, their conflicts within it. As with their individual health care relationships, people with chronic illness often try out many approaches to the health care system over the course of their illness career. The accounts will reveal that these people adapt in astoundingly creative and determined ways so that they may live as well as possible with their illness and its consequences. A description of these strategies and tactics will illuminate a final critical piece in the puzzle of chronic illness experience.

The accounts will illustrate various philosophical and strategic approaches taken by chronically ill people and their families toward obtaining health care inside and outside the existing system. The discussion in this chapter will highlight four themes, each of which represents a common strategic response pattern articulated by many of these patients and families. The first involves generating a philosophical outlook upon the frustrations inherent in the health care system. The second explains the tendency toward increasingly independent decision making with regard to their illness as it progresses over time. The third outlines a variety of tactical maneuvers and strategic skills with which people negotiate their way through the maze of health care. And the fourth reveals the formation of new relationships between fellow travelers in the common quest for those resources fundamental to a rewarding quality of life with chronic illness.

These four patterns of response and resolution reflect an infinite range of tactics and attitudes as the product of an informed analysis of the nature of the health care system. They represent options considered central to a strategic response to the problems inherent in health care for chronic illness. The description will reveal a diversity of strategic options within a common framework of interpretation.

ACQUIESCENCE

For many chronically ill patients and their families, confrontations with the health care system were intolerable. However, from their perspective, continuing the feud between themselves and the system was pointless. As several commented, "You can't change the system." Because of this, finding a philosophical approach with which to address such confrontations was a priority, and the transition from anxiety to a more comfortable attitude was perceived as a step toward health. As one patient explained, "It seems that the more I come to terms with it, the stronger and the healthier I am feeling."

Although accepting the chronic illness itself had been relatively straightforward for many of the men and women in this study, accepting the health care implications was a much more complex matter. While their diseases could generally be attributed to fate or bad luck, their experiences in the health care system were more clearly a product of human failings. Instead of acceptance, therefore, many people developed a philosophical stance that more closely resembled a tolerance or voluntary submission to the system's inherent nature. As one woman expressed it, "I can handle that now, but I don't like it."

Minimizing the Negative

For some people, this attitude of acquiescence involved a determination not to focus on their more negative experiences in health care. At times, such a stance resembled a form of denial, in which the negative experiences they described were afforded minimal importance in the overall experience. One young man concluded, "Except for that one surgeon, and then that one nurse, and that other floor nurse, most of the time it's been really good." For many patients and families, this stance required a reinterpretation of their own previous analysis of the health care system to correct earlier criticisms.

But we are hypocritical, too. We ask . . . that the medical profession does not make mistakes, because it can be very costly, it can cost you your life,

you see. . . . But we are just finding out that they're human—that there are
mistakes being made, right? I mean, we have to adjust to them.

At times, this reinterpretation included finding fault with their own
participation in taking responsibility for their health. At other times, it
consisted of localizing the frustration with health care in a specific
service or professional. For example, one woman, who had expressed
complete lack of faith in all aspects of the health care system on initial
interview, had this to say several months later:

> I don't think I've ever lost total faith in the health care system as a whole.
> You might lose faith in certain individuals. . . . I would say maybe there
> was lots of times I was frustrated with the system, but I wouldn't necessar-
> ily say it was a loss of faith in the system. I always felt there was a light at
> the end of the tunnel, so to speak. . . . You learned how to cope with those
> things and how to adjust to the situation or deal with it, you know, on a
> different level.

While such claims superficially appeared to contradict the analysis
that patients and their families had expressed on other occasions,
careful probing revealed their strategic and functional nature. For example, one patient had been quite convincing in her praise of all that
had happened to her in the health care system. When asked by the
interviewer what would happen if she were given permission to be more
critical, her reply was, "Well, I do that really, but I'm really sneaky
about it." Clearly, she did have negative feelings, but was careful about
when and how she allowed them to surface. For many people, it seemed
far more pleasant to uphold a positive attitude than it was to remain
negative and angry. Thus, denying or minimizing the difficulties seemed
a means by which chronically ill patients and their families could feel
more comfortable with their circumstances in health care.

Emphasizing the Positive

A related strategic approach toward developing an acceptable philosophy was emphasizing the positive side of the overall experience. For
one woman, this was accomplished by focusing on the exceptional
health care professionals she had discovered along the way:

> In some way I began to connect with people within the health care system
> who saw a certain amount of power tripping and controlling happening and

who had found some way to work within that system and yet not perpetuate it. And just in talking to them, or having used their services, it just made me feel that there are some very good people—individuals, working within that system, who have somehow found a way to survive and still do really good work, and not perpetuate the system.

For her, aligning with these wonderful people produced a sense of comradeship in adversity. Another patient looked to her experiences in health care as a potential aid to personal development: "I hope it's going to make me a more loving, more compassionate person when all is said and done."

For many others, negative aspects of the health care experience could be neutralized by recognition of the excellent learning opportunities that they had afforded. For example, some claimed that they had developed a stronger sense of personal responsibility. Others noted a more grounded perspective on life. Still others declared that they had developed a healthy sense of caution and vigilance in their dealings with other people. Thus, negative experiences in health care could be reinterpreted as excellent opportunities to learn and grow.

The accounts revealed that assuaging the negative emotions associated with health care experiences could be an important strategic response for many individuals and families. By developing a coherent philosophical approach to what had happened, these people provided themselves with a comfortable intellectual basis on which to make sense of their ongoing experience.

SELF-RELIANCE

A second strategic response was to develop self-reliance in chronic illness management over time. For many of the men and women interviewed, self-reliance became a strongly held philosophy as well as a tactical response to their health care experience. Relying on themselves rather than on the health care system meant different things to different people. For some, self-reliance meant complete withdrawal from formal health care; for many others, it meant continuing health care, but with radically different motivations and objectives. In either case, however, self-reliance implied becoming well informed and regaining control over decision making with regard to the chronic illness.

Withdrawal

For some patients and families, self-reliance involved complete withdrawal from any involvement in the health care system. For many, withdrawal from health care was motivated by fear of what could happen if they remained involved in an invasive and distorted system. Others withdrew because of a conviction that continuing involvement would inevitably lead to disappointment and greater frustration:

> A few months ago, I said, "To hell with it. We're just going to end up doing all of this by ourselves. Let's not even ask." You get sick of asking. . . . We go through the motions again, and all you can do is you can get disappointed. You get disappointed, then you get mad, and then you say, "To hell with it. We'll just do it ourselves."

And still others explained that participation in health care made them vulnerable to the possibility that some other sign or symptom could launch them back into the medical merry-go-round:

> I've detached myself from that nonsense. And I don't want to be back in their hands, you see, because you lose your self-control, in that sense, and you give it over to them. And they can keep you going for months on end with all kinds of elaborate procedures.

Clearly, for many patients, the investigative process that could be triggered by unnecessary health care involvement could be counterproductive to their physical health as well as to their emotional well-being.

> Here I was, already dealing with a chronic disease process that had climaxed, and still all they were doing was poking at me, and aggravating my bodily state, not really benefiting from any of the medical things that were happening. So I sort of withdrew.

In withdrawing from formal health care entirely, these patients and families had decided that chronic illness care was best managed by themselves and that the health care system would be reserved for dire emergencies. As one woman claimed, "I never see the doctor . . . unless there's a horrible emergency and I'm spurting blood all over the place. Then I might go." By developing techniques for managing both everyday symptoms and acute episodes of their chronic illness, many patients and families were able to avoid involvement with the health care system.

Withdrawing from the health care system was therefore a protective measure by which these chronically ill individuals and their families prevented what they saw as the hazards inherent in allowing the system to take over. For many, it seemed far easier to rely on their own ingenuity than to fight for what they needed in an inhospitable and unsympathetic health care system.

Becoming Well-Informed

Naturally, self-reliance required that chronically ill individuals and their families become highly informed about their options for self-care and illness management. In many cases, this included learning as much as possible about how medical science viewed their particular disease condition. As was noted in earlier discussions, the men and women in this study were remarkable in their range and scope of ingenuity in this regard. From the perspective of these chronically ill individuals and families, obtaining information was key to being less dependent on the opinions of professionals.

Without a scientific background, many people had to struggle to develop confidence that they could use complex and technical information wisely on their own behalf. As one patient explained, "It's funny, you know, all these people . . . are smarter than you are at some particular thing, but there's not one person who is smarter than me about me." However, once they began to effect a shift in confidence, many described an insatiable hunger for knowledge. For many of these people, therefore, continued involvement with the health care system became important as one of many possible sources for the information required to be successfully self-reliant.

As they became aware of a greater variety of information sources and the contradictions inherent in them, these patients and families were forced to develop a critical approach to information. While a few engaged in formal systematic study, many described a sort of constant comparative analytic process by which they interpreted each new piece of formal knowledge in the light of what they knew from their own experience. From their perspective, self-reliance was dependent not only on obtaining essential information, but also on learning to appraise it critically before applying it to personal decision making. Thus, the self-reliance described by these chronically ill individuals and their families was the outcome of excellent information and critical appraisal of its applicability to their particular circumstances.

Regaining Control

For the patients and families in this study, a commitment to self-reliance grew out of gradual recognition that they were, in fact, the experts with regard to their own disease and its repercussions. The inevitable conclusion that they were the best judge of their own unique circumstances was a difficult discovery for many. It required a clear interpretation of the limits of health care in the case of chronic illnesses. It also required that the limits of people within the health care system be acknowledged. As one patient noted, "There are a lot of people in the health care system that don't know what they're doing, and they don't care either. And I can do a better job than they can."

Regaining control required that those with chronic illness become confident that their own understanding about general well-being was as valid as any clinical or technical expertise for making chronic illness decisions. Once achieved, such confidence created a sense of harmony and balance in lives that had previously been tossed and turned by the events of health care. It gave them strength in the knowledge that they were avoiding harm and promoting health by taking actions consistent with an informed interpretation of health and well-being. Their descriptions of how it felt to be back in control revealed a renewed sense of order and logic in illness management, regardless of whether formal health care was involved.

For some patients and families, being in control meant avoiding medical care as much as possible. As an alternative, many managed their illness through life-style manipulation. For example, one woman took up swimming; eliminated caffeine, sugar, and tobacco; and began taking vitamins in order to avoid medical treatment for her arthritis. In other cases, regaining control meant determining not only the conditions under which formal health care was appropriate but also the type of health care that would be tolerated. In this way, it allowed continuing participation in health care with a coherent plan for the predictable future. As one woman explained, "It's as though I did not ever want to be caught out at that again in terms of my own innocence and my own ignorance." It also allowed for the possibility of using multiple services that would ordinarily be considered incompatible. As one patient expressed it, "I see myself with a foot either side of the fence."

For some patients and families, regaining control meant outright noncompliance with unacceptable aspects of a treatment plan that was otherwise acceptable. In one such instance, after considerable research and soul-searching, a mother decided to take her child off a PKU diet: "It's really hard. The doctors look at it from their point of view, and I'm looking at it from a mother's point of view." Although they often described such noncompliance as a difficult decision, many explained how it freed them from the far more difficult problems associated with giving up control: "You know, you're the one that has to live with it, not them. They go along and do their work, and they don't realize how it is." In their view, noncompliance proved that they had liberated themselves from earlier fears of what would happen if they defied the authorities. Whether they avoided professional health care as much as possible or continued to used it selectively, the important issue for these patients and families was their own ability to retain control over the course of events in their illness management. As one informant rejoiced, "I'm in control, and it feels great."

According to the informants in this study, self-reliance in chronic illness management was a major test of the competence and judgment of patients and families. Despite awareness of the possibility that they might guess wrong, these people were confident that the strategy was in and of itself beneficial. One woman explained, "It's still kind of scary. But at least, if I'm going to die, it's going to be because I've made the mistake. . . . I'm not going to wait for some doctor to lay it on me."

Thus, the self-reliance described by these people was a philosophical and strategic response to the political and ideological problems they had encountered in health care. It offered them a range of options and freed them from many of the hazards associated with dependence on the health care system. By defining themselves as self-reliant, these chronically ill individuals and families took charge of their own lives. They used their own judgments about health and well-being as the standard against which to decide what health care they would accept and what they would reject.

STRATEGIC DEPENDENCE

In apparent contrast to the self-reliant approach, many patients and families articulated strategies by which they could manipulate or enhance the health care on which they felt dependent. For various reasons, ranging from psychological dependence on the expertise of professionals to practical dependence on resources accessible only through cooperation with those professionals, some chronically ill individuals and their families conceded to utter dependence upon the health care system. However, rather than maintaining the uncritical dependence that had created so much frustration, these people generated numerous creative strategies to increase the consistency with which they could get what they really needed from the system.

In general, strategic dependence reflected a combination of assertiveness and manipulation. As one patient said, "You play the system." As with self-reliance, strategic dependence required that patients and families begin to take responsibility for their health care encounters, and depended upon their ability to make accurate judgments about what they needed from the health care system. As one man explained, "The difference is that I now approach the traditional medical profession with an eye to getting mechanical, technical responses that I already know are appropriate."

In this discussion, four types of strategic dependence will be described, ranging from subtle manipulation of the goodwill of health care staff to outright challenges to the social order of health care. Each strategy will reveal a means by which chronically ill individuals and their families manipulate a system upon which they feel dependent. Thus, the discussion will demonstrate the remarkable variety of creative tactics by which these people resolved some of their most serious difficulties with the health care system.

Generating Goodwill

From the perspective of many chronically ill individuals and families, an intelligent response to some of the human frailties in health care was to create a sense of goodwill among the health care providers. By being sociable, polite, grateful, and respectful, many people found that they could exert considerable control over their interactions in health care. One man, for example, explained the importance of keeping track of names so as to personalize his greetings to a large number of health care workers. As he explained, "I know that if you don't go out of your way to try to recognize a person that's being some help to you, it isn't long before that help might dry up." Similarly, a woman commented that, by being a "good patient," her brother earned preferential treatment during his frequent hospitalizations. Thus, strategic adoption of the "good patient" role seemed to serve these people well in their health care interactions.

Overt demonstration of respect for the professionals was also identified as a way to generate goodwill. Sometimes, this was accomplished by strategic use of questions designed to reveal admiration for the professional's knowledge, while at the same time providing hints of the patient's desires. At other times, such respect was demonstrated through exhibiting compliance with the prescribed treatment. According to one mother, compliance provided an excellent way of generating goodwill from the professionals at her clinic. "I guess we're the kind of people, we do what they tell us to do. They know we're—they call it compliant."

By showing respect and by demonstrating personal concern for the people administering their health care, many patients and families believed they were able to set themselves apart from the general population and obtain a favored position as good patients. Thus, from their perspective, such a strategy was an excellent means for maintaining certain services upon which they felt dependent.

Monitoring Professionals

Another form of strategic dependence involved carefully monitoring the behavior and decisions of the health professionals involved in their care. Such monitoring revealed concern that professionals were not always 100% attentive to their responsibilities. As one woman explained, "That doctor is going to see hundred of intestines, but this is my only one and I want to make sure that what he's going to tell me to do is what's really going to be best for me."

In many cases, monitoring the professionals included maintaining careful documentation of all health care decisions and actions. In other instances, it involved seeing for themselves the bases upon which professionals made decisions. For example, one mother recalled sneaking a peek at her son's medical record: "I know the doctors, if they knew I did that, would just about shit bricks, you know. I mean, that's sort of like sacred papers." From her point of view, being able to see the record for herself provided a sense of security.

By keeping track of their treatment over time, many patients and families were able to ensure that they were not lost in the bureaucratic shuffle. One woman explained that she booked her appointments three months in advance to be sure she was not forgotten. A young man recalled telephoning the doctor from time to time during non-acute phases to remind him to order blood work. Such strategies often allowed patients and families to circumvent some of the more frustrating bureaucratic deficiencies. Thus, monitoring the professionals and the services they provided allowed them to take steps toward ensuring the continuity and the quality of health care.

Another form of monitoring described by many patients and families was surreptitiously evaluating professional recommendations prior to following them. As one woman explained, she would look up drug prescriptions in the pharmacopoeia. Another telephoned respected hospitals across the continent to inquire about their policies with regard to certain treatments. And a third compared the suggestions of other professionals and patients in addition to reading about the problem. Sometimes this strategy also included checking up on the credentials of the professionals and their services. For example, one woman claimed to have investigated infection rates prior to selecting a hospital for surgery.

Beyond these tactics, patients and families described numerous additional forms of monitoring. One man described keeping track of the insurable visits to various therapists to be sure that he obtained the maximum permitted in any calendar year. A woman described pumping nurses for information so that she could judge their opinions of doctors. And many patients and families described a sense of vigilance during times of intense health care involvement, such as hospitalization. By monitoring what was happening, these people felt that they were doing something to ensure the best possible health care for themselves or their loved one. As one patient explained, "I wouldn't want to just sit there and have them come and do things to her, and me not know why."

By documenting their own care, by checking out the credentials or the recommendations of certain professionals against other sources of information, and by maintaining a vigilant stance, these patients and families felt that they were able to exert considerable control over the quality of their health care.

Withholding Consent

While dependent patients could rarely dictate their treatment, the possibility of withholding consent for aspects of health care was a powerful playing card. The accounts reveal that many patients and families considered the option of saying "No" to be a critical defensive strategy for those dependent on health care. The idea that they could refuse to cooperate with what the health care system expected of them was a remarkably liberating discovery for many patients and families. Once they recognized the power of withholding consent, many people were able to eliminate some of the more frustrating aspects of the health care experience.

The accounts of withholding consent revealed that it could be usefully applied in many different contexts. Many described refusing medication unless the rationale for taking it was acceptable. Others recalled learning to refuse diagnostic procedures. As one man commented, "An X-ray that's only going to satisfy their curiosity, to me is a waste of money, and a waste of my pain, and stuff." In some cases, withholding consent reflected open conflict. One woman's story of a male physician who insisted on performing a vaginal exam illustrates: "I said, 'You may think you're hot shit, but I don't, and you're not touching me,' you know. And then, of course, I got treated like a piece of shit! But I just refused to give in to it." In contrast, many instances of withholding consent were handled with subtlety and finesse. One patient, for example, used the hint that she might refuse to cooperate as a tactic to obtain a special favor: "Myasthenia is quite rare—and he wanted me to do a seminar to his students. . . . And I said 'Fine'—if he could get me a pass to use the medical library."

In each of these cases, actually or potentially withholding consent was a means by which patients and families remained in control over their care, in spite of being quite dependent on the system. From their perspective, the realization that they could refuse care was a critical turning point, enabling them to stand up for their own rights as consumers. By merely deciding that their consent could be withheld at any time for any reason, these patients and families were able to regain a sense of control over their health care situations.

> It's been one of the hardest things to learn. Like I don't have to take shit and abuse any more. You know, I don't have to be treated like a piece of shit from anybody—including doctors and nurses. You know, I have control in that. I don't have to jump into a victim [stance], and I don't have to take it. You know, I can stand up for me, and my rights, and who I am as a person . . . I'm sorry, but I refuse to give anybody that control over me.

Thus, for those dependent on health care in chronic illness, the threat of withholding consent was powerful ammunition in their confrontations with the health care system.

Challenging the Social Order

At the polar extreme from the strategy of generating goodwill was the realization, articulated by several patients and families, that they could wield a great deal of power by upsetting the normal social order within health care. In contrast to manipulating the system by being "good" patients, these people found the "bad" patient role to be equally strategic.

Departing from the usual social order in health care, some patients and families believed that the threat of a lawsuit would make it difficult for professionals to refuse reasonable requests outright. While none admitted to outright threats or actions in this regard, many considered the fact that they might have a legal case as a useful bargaining tool. Similarly, some patients and families challenged the social order in health care by lodging formal complaints within the bureaucracy itself. For example, one man admitted that he often reported staff who were not treating him as he expected to be treated. And one woman described registering a successful complaint about the filthy conditions in her hospital unit. Thus, for several of these patients and families, the options of launching a lawsuit or filing a formal complaint were empowering possibilities.

In addition, many of the patients and families discovered that overtly expressing anger was an extremely effective challenge to the social order in health care. In some instances, people described being aggressive with health care professionals. As one mother explained, "Unless I throw my weight around, and unless I am alert to whatever, it's not necessarily assured that [my child's] needs are going to get met." Through such techniques as blocking doorways, raising their voices, and refusing to leave waiting rooms until they were seen, several people were able to demonstrate their anger with positive effect. In other cases, people described the benefits of such extreme expressions as temper tantrums and creating disturbances. As one man explained:

> [My wife] and I get better things for [our child] now only because we've learned how to beat the system. You go in there and you scream your guts out and tell them what you want. And after a while they get scared of you that you're going to do something bizarre, and they give you what you want (*laugh*).... You get to the point where you're so goddamned mad it doesn't matter anyway. You don't feel like you have to maintain some kind of degree of sanity. After awhile, you can go absolutely nutso and it's kind of a relief anyway.

Because anger was not consistent with the expected patient role, it could be sufficiently disrupting to give the advantage to the chronically ill individual and family. Thus, for some brave people, calculated departures from the noncritical, compliant, quiet role expected of them could be an effective strategy in retaining some control, despite dependence on the health care system.

What has been conceptualized here as strategic dependence is therefore a collection of tools and tactics by which people sought to increase their advantage and retain as much control as possible while remaining involved in health care. Although the tactics described ranged from subtle and unassuming to much more overt and violent, they were all predicated on two basic principles. The first was that complete dependence on the health care system was unhealthy. The second was that no one but themselves would take responsibility for the whole process. For these chronically ill people and their families, being clever, vigilant, and outspoken were therefore essential tools of the trade.

MAKING CONNECTIONS

A final theme in the accounts of how chronically ill patients and their families responded to the health care system reveals the critical importance of making connections with people of similar experience. In this discussion, the efforts of those living with chronic illness to find, create, or sustain networks among themselves will be the focus. Alliances between people living with chronic illness ranged from spontaneous discoveries of common experience to formal societies and organizations. In this study, the vast majority of informants reported some degree of cooperative involvement for the purpose of dealing with the difficulties inherent in obtaining health care for a chronic illness. These formal and informal contacts were described as having two central purposes: information and support.

Information Networks

The chronically ill individuals and families in this study described a number of self-help groups, nonprofit organizations, and related networks whose primary objective was to share information about the chronic illness and its management. The accounts of their participation in such networks revealed that these patients and families valued belonging to a larger social phenomenon, sometimes referred to as "the consumer movement."

Most of the informants made their initial contacts with such agencies for the specific purpose of obtaining information deemed essential for illness management. Networks often included newsletters, public meetings, and formalized societies, each of which had an educational function. The information imparted through these means ranged from basic patient information to an analysis of current research developments and medical breakthroughs. Several informants claimed that becoming familiar with the research provided the feeling that they were doing something constructive. As one woman remarked, "I take a lot of heart from the statistics." However, what professionals had to say did not always match the patient's and the family's experience. According to one woman, "A lot of the invited doctors who stood up and spoke, spoke whereof they did not know."

Although information networks provided an efficient means of obtaining the most recent technical, research, and clinical information applicable to their particular health problem, they also confronted people with extremely painful realities. One woman's story illustrates:

> I went to the national convention last year.... And some of the things are really upsetting to me. Like I went back to the room and I just wanted to cry. Like I just couldn't deal with them. I don't want to think about this happening, you know—people's stories . . . I don't want to hear. I mean, if they say, when we have an executive meeting and the clinic liaison, three times this year, said, "We lost another child this week." I mean, you just look around the room, and . . . I can see people visibly tense up. They don't want to know.

Another woman reported that she found herself feeling too sorry for other people she met through participation in such networks. "I generally can't sleep after, you know. It brings it too much to the surface." Thus, such access to information could be simultaneously comforting and acutely disturbing for the chronically ill patients and families.

Beyond seeking information on their own behalf, a great many of the men and women in this study had active involvement with disseminating information to other patients and families. As will be recalled from earlier discussions, many had experienced difficulty obtaining information about their own health problem during the early adjustment period. As a result, many believed that they could make an important contribution to those with less experience as well as to future patients and families. As one woman explained, it was satisfying to help meet the needs of newer patients and families:

Whenever I hear of anybody that's got Crohn's or colitis, I'll either send them literature, or say, "Listen, if you want someone to talk to, any time, just phone me up." Whenever I run into people, or somebody knows somebody, I just want to help them. Just so that they don't have the troubles of finding doctors that we went through.

The work of disseminating information involved a number of tasks that were themselves quite demanding of these patients and families. One mother, for example, found herself giving public lectures. She recalled, "It wasn't easy for me to get up in front of the public. It's years since I have done that. But I had my notes, and I got up shakily, and I got into it quite well." Others became involved in organizing meetings, hosting lectures, or preparing newsletters. The activities involved often brought people into contact with a symbolic community of others interested in similar issues. One woman described how exciting it had been to learn from a Californian Scleroderma society that there were five other patients in her area. Within a year, she had created a local branch and attracted 43 members. Others described extensive international connections they had made in the process of communicating with other disease-related consumer organizations. Finally, some of the informants in this study envisioned their role as extending to active fund-raising for the purpose of stimulating new research that might empower patients and treat the disease.

The work involved in such information networks was often complex, sophisticated, and demanding. Participation in such activities reflected an exhaustive commitment for some people, as one woman revealed: "It's been a huge part of my life for 3 years. Like I am totally involved in anything that they're doing. They always know that they can count on me, that I'll be there." Whether their involvement was confined to obtaining information or they became involved in the process of disseminating information to others, information networks helped chronically ill individuals and their families to understand their health care experience in a larger context and, therefore, to do something constructive about it.

Support Groups

Many patients and families also talked of their experiences in groups whose primary objective was social support for those with a particular illness. According to many of these men and women, hospital and clinic waiting rooms provided their first such experience with peer support:

The parents' lounges are mini support groups on your own. You've got everybody with every problem in there, and if somebody sees somebody crying, there's always somebody will go over and put an arm around and say, "Hey, what's the matter?" If somebody has a successful thing happen, everybody, you know, feels their joy for them.

In many cases, the alliances that were formed in such circumstances created the initial inspiration to set up a more formal support group.

As seemed evident in the accounts of what made information networks so popular, many of those living with chronic illness felt a burning desire to make contact with others who had encountered similar experiences. One woman recalled that attending a public lecture had been her first exposure to others with her disease:

Even though it's a lecture, and there's no personal talking going on between the people that are there, or with the person that lectures, this was a help to me to know that there were other people in the room like me.

Another woman remembered a similar urgency to connect with other patients and families. "The first meeting I went to . . . I stood in the parking lot for about an hour and a half in the cold (*laugh*) because I wanted to talk to someone so badly." For many, such contact with others in similar circumstances helped them feel that they were not alone.

The obvious appeal of such groups was the probability that they would find others who could truly appreciate what they were living through. In such support groups, social differences often paled in comparison to the common bond that fellow patients and family members shared: "We're from different walks of life, we're totally, totally different, except that we share something really common—we have the same disease." Further, these men and women found the support group to represent a context in which their stories about their disease and about its health care consequences would be believed.

If I told them any of these stupid things that had happened, they'll understand. They'll believe, and they'll understand, even if they don't say anything. I know they know that I'm not making this whole thing up. And they all have their own ugly stories.

Besides understanding their situation, support group members could offer valuable suggestions for coping with the disease and its consequences. From the perspective of many patients and families, the ideas of others prevented them from having to learn everything the hard way. As one man explained, "Why reinvent the wheel? . . . Why should I have to take a year or 2 years to figure that out for myself?" Further, they provided an alternative to formal health care consultation in decision making about the illness. As one young mother recalled, "If one of the kids were sick we'd all phone each other first, and say, 'Well, what do you think?' " In this way, support groups helped patients and families understand their own experiences with a greater sense of perspective than they had been able to sustain alone. Thus, as one man concluded, "Support groups are a big asset to every chronic disease."

The accounts of what made support groups important to so many patients and families in this study, however, did not merely reflect their role in support for living with a chronic disease. More important, according to many of the informants, they provided a source of support and insight for dealing with the health care system. Often, the knowledge that their frustrations were not unique was quite a revelation, as one father recalled:

> A lot of stuff I heard had to do with the same kind of frustrations we were talking about tonight, with doctors not telling them what's wrong, and the health care system. . . . I was quite surprised, because I didn't realize that there were so many that felt the same. You know, out of 12 guys, pretty well all of them expressed the same frustrations!

Such groups therefore helped people develop constructive responses to the shared problems they had encountered in health care. Further, they provided people with access to essential information about available facilities and resources that they had been unable to obtain otherwise. As one man explained, his wife "found out a lot of her things by going to the morning bullshit sessions that the wives have when the kids are getting therapy." Support groups also bolstered people's courage to be more critical in health care encounters. As one woman noted, she would not have thought to ask for photocopies of written reports until learning from other parents in her support group that it was possible. Finally, such groups also helped patients and families develop confidence that their own judgments were no less valid than were those of professionals. Thus, for many people living with chronic illness, support groups were an extraordinarily valuable resource for learning how to cope with some of the most difficult issues in their health care experience.

Although support groups were immensely important to these informants, many were actively discouraged from such involvements by their professional health care providers. Typically, the professionals failed to mention the existence of support groups, even for patients and families who openly expressed a need for such support. One woman recalled her amazement at discovering how resistant the health care system was toward providing patients with this sort of information:

> I've often said that to the Arthritis Society, "Why didn't you tell me that there were support groups?" And they said, "Well, we just don't have that facility within our organization to communicate that to you." And I said, "Why don't you start doing that now? Why don't you start handing out information and telling people?" But nobody hands that out and they still don't.

Similarly, one mother remembered intense resistance from physicians when a group of parents had tried to start a support group:

> They don't want PKU parents talking to each other—that's my very strong belief—because we compare. . . . And at one of our meetings, we did have the doctors come out to the meeting, and it was like they were like politicians. When you asked them a question, you never did get the answer to the question. . . . And I don't know if it was because they didn't know, or they didn't want us to know, and they didn't like us comparing the kids. And it was almost as if they thought we were stupid.

From the perspective of these chronically ill individuals and families, this same resistance was evident in such decisions as refusing to grant meeting space for support groups, withholding mailing lists on the pretense of patient confidentiality, and even openly criticizing support group leaders as disturbed and disruptive individuals.

Support groups, therefore, offered those living with chronic illness the comfort of knowing others with similar health problems, but also represented a challenge to the authority of the health care system. As some professionals clearly suspected, patients and families found support groups to be a source of fuel for their criticism of the health care system as well as for their noncompliance with its expectations. Through their involvement with information and support networks, many chronically ill patients and their families were able to forge connections with their peers to respond to those shared frustrations. The accounts reveal that such connections addressed not only the immediate effects of the illness itself, but also the health care consequences. Thus, the consumer movement described by these informants represented a critical social force in direct response to problems in health care.

DISCUSSION

Following upon descriptions of the confrontations chronically ill people and their families have in the health care system and the interpretations they make of such confrontations, this chapter has reviewed some of the creative and colorful strategies with which such individuals and families respond. It has surveyed philosophical strategies designed to make the best of a bad situation and to take on as much personal responsibility as possible, as well as tactical strategies for manipulating the system as far as possible, individually and with the strength of numbers.

The various strategic responses revealed in these accounts are all represented in the scholarly literature in some form. Such actions as withdrawal from health care, control-seeking, and exaggerated independence in chronic illness tend to be regarded as rather counterproductive within the health care literature (Arpin, Fitch, Browne, & Corey, 1988; Black, Dornan, & Allegrante, 1986; Viney, 1983). Usually, such responses are explained as indications of the powerlessness patients feel in the face of a chronic condition, rather than as evidence of their power in devising rational responses to an intolerant health care system (Mechanic, 1979a; Nordstrom & Lubkin, 1990). Further, the central importance of information and support groups is also widely acknowledged in the literature. However, the meaning that such cooperative networks have in the lives of chronically ill people is usually understood as information and support with regard to the disease rather than its care (Dallery, 1983; Lord, 1989; Williams, 1989).

If the response patterns of individual patients or families in this study were to be considered separately, each would reveal threads of the categories described here, and no two would be identical. How each person living with chronic illness responds to the common problems seems dependent upon a range of complex factors inherent in the illness experience. Some patients and families can control their symptoms and experience a reasonable quality of life without resorting to professional health care; for others, withdrawal from supportive services would mean death or further serious disability. Some patients and families gain confidence about their illness and its management by making successful judgments over time; for others, an early weak judgment may have a lasting effect on self-confidence. Finally, some patients and families find support inside or outside the formal health care system that enables them to resolve their major conflicts early in the game; for others, supports are never found and the conflicts never resolved. The variables of symptom control, confidence, and support, therefore, seem critical in determining the unique pattern of response that each individual and family creates.

Despite variations in technique, however, the many strategic responses described by these patients and families follow a similar course through dependence, to anger and, finally, to a feeling of control:

> I've gone full circle. I've gone from at the beginnings being, "Help me, help me. You've got to help me. I know you can help me." And thinking, okay, here's the doctors and the medical profession, okay, they'll help you. Don't worry about it, you'll be okay. They're going to do something for you. And then getting into it more, changing to, "Who are you trying to fool? You can't help me. You guys are just making me worse and you're lying to me . . . " [And then] to being more open. And when they realized that I turned that way, my attitude became like that, they would be more open to me. It's like they realized where I was coming from, and what I knew.

In examining the coping of the chronically ill and their families in this light, the similarities seem more prominent than the differences. Such apparently contrasting coping styles as compliance and noncompliance, politeness and rudeness, independence and dependence, can all be understood as means toward a similar end: exerting an influence over what happens in health care encounters. In this manner, the accounts suggest that we can no more infer their analysis from their coping behavior than we can assume their prognosis from their physical appearance.

From the perspective of the men and women in this study, the range of rational responses to the insults of health care for chronic illness seems infinite. Spirited and imaginative strategies clearly enable many people with chronic illness to live well. However, as the accounts have revealed, this often occurs in spite of rather than because of the health care they receive. By distinguishing coping with health care from coping with illness itself, this discussion has brought the patients' and the families' interpretation of their own coping strategies to center stage. In so doing, it has challenged us to take another look at our interpretation of what we think coping with chronic illness is all about. When we read in the chronic illness literature, therefore, that adaptations are required, that there is emotional distress, and that support must be developed, it seems no longer acceptable to assume that these are all factors wrought by the ravages of disease upon the person. Rather, we ought to interpret these as equally applicable to the violation that ongoing involvement in the health care system seems to unleash upon those with chronic illnesses and their families.

The Course Ahead

The chronic illness experience has been conceptualized in preceding chapters as a complex social phenomenon emerging from factors inherent in a disease, in a society, and in a health care system. Uncovering the layers of the meaning of chronic illness within the lives of those afflicted, it has become increasingly apparent that the chronic illness experience cannot be fully appreciated without an analysis of the health care context in which it takes place. The patients and families whose stories have contributed to this analysis make a convincing argument in support of the conclusion that their thoughts, their actions, and their adaptations are all profoundly influenced by their experiences in trying to find a way through an ideologically and bureaucratically complex health care system. In order to understand why chronically ill people behave in the way that they do, the implications of health care must be factored into the analysis.

Despite experiences within the health care system that range from the frustrating and exhausting to the horrifying, demoralizing, and dehumanizing, the infinite adaptability of the human psyche and intellect helps these people find creative ways with which to minimize the negative repercussions of health care for chronic illness. Because they must, they find a way through the maze and often accomplish remarkable successes in their lives. However, the anger and distrust with which they view the health care system do not disappear. There is evidence that, nationally and internationally, chronically ill people and their families are forming relationships, gaining knowledge, and accumulating legal and political strength. They are, increasingly, a force that may shape the society of our future.

In the face of this growing population of critical and distrustful chronically ill individuals and their families, the health care system lumbers along, recreating the same flawed structures and perfecting the same errors. While there is widespread acknowledgment of problems in health care, one finds little agreement on what ought to be changed. Typically, Band-Aid solutions such as more money, more beds, and more doctors are proposed. What these would do to solve the problems of chronic illness is rarely considered. As seems clear to critics both in the consumer movement and in health care analysis, the problems inherent in the health care of today demand radical reform.

In this final chapter, some visions of the course ahead in health care will be proposed. The discussion will note some of the possibilities put forth by chronically ill patients and their families in the course of their analysis of health care, and will complement these with reference to scholarly proposals recorded in the critical health care literature. Although literature on the Canadian health care system is most directly applicable to this analysis, the ideas of those writing about other health care systems will not be disregarded. While there are obvious national differences, this discussion will draw upon some of the deeper, and perhaps more telling, similarities. Thus, through an examination of what some people think might make a significant difference, a portrait of a health care system more appropriate to chronic illness will begin to take shape.

In contrast to the tightly coherent academic disciplines that confine much of the scholarly literature, the interpretations of chronically ill patients and their families cross economic, social, political, and philosophical boundaries to form opinions about what ought to change and how change ought to be orchestrated. From their perspective, each contradiction in health care is entangled in others, each problem in health care is a piece of a larger problem, and each solution in health care is, therefore, dependent on other solutions. The discussion of these questions here will be organized into three interrelated but conceptually distinguishable themes drawn from the interpretations of patients and families who participated in this study. Thus, the analysis of the course ahead will include opinions about what ought to change in the general domains of health care organization, biomedical ideology, and, finally, social policy.

For many of the patients and families in this study, the metaphor of technology gone wild depicts the investment structure, intrinsic motivation, and authority patterns characteristic of the problems in the health care system today. Their visions of the future ahead emerge in snippets of analysis and are never presented as the complete picture.

Indeed, the humility reflected in the academic literature suggests that the complete picture is beyond the capacity of most scholars as well. Among those who put forth their ideas, there are few who confidently claim to have answers, and even they are quickly discredited by equally compelling but completely incompatible proposals. Like the opinions of the scholars, the interpretations of the chronically ill will not provide final answers to the raging questions that concern us here. However, they may help to steer us on a course that makes discovery possible.

HEALTH CARE ORGANIZATION

As the accounts of the individuals and families who participated in this study reveal, the organization of chronic illness services within the existing health care delivery system is complex, inefficient, and frustrating. From their perspective, major changes in the organization of health care delivery could reduce some of the problems that arise from the current chaotic situation.

While they may have application in acute illness and emergency care, many of the bureaucratic policies embedded in health care seem archaic and destructive in the context of chronic illness. According to the chronically ill, the typical rules of hospitalization, referral systems, and access to information are particularly frustrating:

> The one thing I would want . . . for the nurses to understand is that you have the right to say, "I'm not taking that pill," and accept it instead of being angry at me, because now they're going to waste time calling the doctor, and it's going to put them behind their work load, or whatever, you know—the dietitian isn't going to throw her hands up in the air because the patient has refused their food, you know. I would like to be able to carry through what I know I would do, and have the nurse who's taking care of me understand where I'm coming from, and realize I have a right to do that, because it is my body.

From their point of view, such rules often exist only to maintain the authority structure within institutions and cannot be justified on the basis of clinical or social welfare interests. They reflect the assumption that patients are mere resources to feed the system, rather than the intended beneficiaries of its existence. Further, as patients and families point out, such standardizations are inherently abusive where human well-being is concerned. From their perspective, the principle of individualizing care cannot be ignored if quality of life is the ultimate goal. One young man's plea for flexibility was echoed by many of his peers:

> Well, if they just used their heads sometimes . . . rather than just going straight by the book, kind of thing. Just a little common sense would go a long way—like listening to the patient. And, you know, the doctor isn't always right. Every time he says something, it doesn't mean it's gospel.

Thus, patients and families propose that many rules ought to be reconsidered for their applicability in chronic illness and modified accordingly.

Another aspect of health care organization that requires adjustment, according to patients and their families, is the coordination of various health care services. The chronically ill are often afflicted in multiple organ systems, necessitating the involvement of multiple professionals as consultants and advisers. Rarely does any professional orchestrate the input from these various directions, and, in most instances, the patient and family are left to try to sort out the conflicting and confusing advice on their own.

> You've got all these symptoms, and they're happening months apart and sometimes a year apart. Something different will happen in some other part of your body. And you're going to a throat specialist, and you're going to an ear specialist, and you're going to a foot specialist, and you're going to a heart specialist. And you need someone to put all of that together.

The individual who controls access to the rest of the services, usually the general practitioner, is often inaccessible except by appointment and in person. To complicate the problem, general practitioners refer patients to specialists when questions about the illness exceed their narrow scope of expertise. In such instances, both generalist and specialist can then abdicate responsibility for coordinating the patient's care. According to Mechanic (1987), such circumstances absolve physicians from feeling responsible. The stories of patients and families reveal many instances of participating in a merry-go-round of referral, only to discover that it was an exercise in futility; one more person confirms that the problem exists, and no one takes any responsibility for doing anything toward alleviating it. One man spoke for many when he envisioned a system in which all parties actually communicate with each other to define a coordinated plan for the patient:

I'd love to see a surgeon, a gastroenterologist, a dietitian possibly, and maybe the head nurse, or something, plus maybe your mother, your father, your relative, your wife, whatever, sitting down there and all sort of going, "What are the options?" And then everybody knows what the other one thinks, what the options are, what the patient thinks, what he's able to cope with, kind of thing, and then go from there. That'd be great. That's what I'd love to see.

An important element missing from health care for chronic illness is, therefore, the coordinating function.

A related problem is derived from the influence that reimbursement practices are believed to have on the clinical decisions of professionals. Office visits, often necessitating significant energy expenditure, discomfort, and frustration for the patient, are the price of the physician's agreement to needed drugs and services. Patients and families seem well aware that telephone consultations suffice under two conditions— that the physician trusts the patient's claim without visual confirmation, and that the physician is willing to forgo the remuneration that would have accrued from the office visit. Since these conditions represent humility and altruism in the extreme among practitioners, the telephone referral is rarely possible. Thus, medical offices are clogged with people who know their own needs but must have an authoritative confirmation before they can gain access to services.

The contention that remuneration schemes influence clinical decision making is also expressed in the professional literature. Luft (1986), for example, believes that economic incentives bias physicians toward laboratory tests and therapeutic procedures in contrast to taking time with patients. Further, he reports that remuneration derived from supporting high technology may explain the tendency of many physicians toward highly technological clinical options. In an analysis of various payment schemes and their influence on professional behavior, Glaser (1986) reports that fee-for-service systems, such as those in nearly every developed country today, provide little incentive for the types of logical solutions that these patients propose. Thus, the suspicion of patients that their lives are frustrated by procedures whose sole justification is to remunerate physicians seems well founded.

Although routine repetitive tasks such as writing prescriptions and making referrals create few intrinsic rewards in general medical practice (Ben-Sira, 1988), they are far more lucrative than are other options such as counseling patients. Because doctors are notoriously too busy to listen to the concerns of patients, to provide emotional support, and to participate in the problem solving required to manage daily living, many patients and families believe that they are not the appropriate professional to serve as system gatekeepers in the case of chronic illness:

> In the Middle Ages, they had court doctors, right? Even at that time, the court doctor would look after one aristocrat, and he would find out the history of this person, and he would study it. That was his life study, right? But if you put through 150 people a day, I mean, what are you going to find out?

Many patients and families have found that other professionals, generally but not exclusively nurses, have a strong grasp on what the system has to offer and how it may be applied to suit individual health care needs. However, they usually lack the authority to make recommendations without a physician's approval. Further, they do not "belong" to the patient in the way that a physician does, and are generally understood to be inaccessible once the service to which they are attached is no longer required. From the perspective of many patients and families, therefore, the ideal primary clinician for the organization of their health care would be one with an interest in problem solving from a broad basis, one who is accessible for telephone consultation, and one who can procure necessary health care services on their behalf:

> I think the first and foremost thing that I would like is somebody that I could call on the phone and say, "This is what's happening, you know. Should I bring her in? Should I not bring her in?" you know. Somebody that would be available just to do some of that troubleshooting at an initial stage, without having to make it a big deal. . . . I think that would be worth its weight in gold.

In their opinion, access to such a person would ease a tremendous amount of pressure on the system as a whole. Patients and families use such terms as *ombudsman for health, go-between,* and *advocate* to explain how they imagine such a professional could act on their behalf, to steer them through the system and help them make sense of it all. In the professional literature, advocates of such a role term it a *mediator* role (LaFargue, 1985). In the words of one patient, "You almost need somebody to educate people as to how to work with the medical system."

For many patients and families, the political struggles between health care professions are detrimental to chronic illness care. Because physicians are the professionals with formal authority, but the nurses are often the ones that have listened to the patient and family at length, chronically ill people commonly find themselves party to conflict between nurses and doctors with regard to their illness management. The accounts on which this study was based reveal countless instances of nurses openly contesting the decisions or actions of physicians involved in the patients' care. Such instances convince many chronically ill patients that nurses often know better than doctors what would be an appropriate course of action. Thus, they propose that measures to reduce the somewhat misleading status differential (and salary) between nurses and doctors would be in the interests of the chronically ill. For example, some expect that improved conditions for nurses might help improve their stature in health care:

> I think I've seen, to use a hackneyed phrase, that nurses are evolving. And no longer are they the handmaiden of the physician, who certainly spoke down to them, and there's no question about that. And they've got a long way to go. . . . If nurses received better pay in return for their work, there wouldn't be such a shortage. And I think at the same time, you'd have to raise the standards and qualifications and things and give them some more responsibility.

Others propose that nurses ought to become more politically demanding to effect some of these essential changes in their relations with doctors:

> If they want office workers, secretaries, whatever, why do they educate them? Why drag them through 4 years of looking after the sick, and then pen them up in an office. . . . And, another thing I think about nurses, I think they better put their spines up, and start talking back to the doctors. Because the nurses, in the majority of cases, the nurses know a hell of a lot more than the doctor does.

The literature contains ample evidence that this view is shared by many scholars and health care analysts (McKinlay & Stoeckle, 1988). For example, Lynaugh (1988) believes that modern health delivery systems tend to deprive chronically ill patients of the services that nurses could provide by restricting reimbursement to those factors of interest to physicians. She further suggests that nurses have subsidized excessively high physician incomes by remaining on the economic margins of the health care system.

Another feature of health care organization of great concern to chronically ill patients and families is the degree to which error and incompetence are tolerated. From their perspective, protection of the autonomy of professionals allows insensitive, cruel, and dehumanizing acts to be justified from a clinical perspective. In the absence of formal channels through which to express their criticisms, these patients and families rely on support groups and informal networks to advise others about whom to avoid and whom to trust. However, they are adamant that there ought to be mechanisms within the structure of health care delivery for weeding out the most serious offenders. In their view, this would require a shift in the attitude of professionals toward recognizing that such abuses really do take place in the name of clinical privilege. A similar view is also argued in the critical professional literature. For example, Bosk's (1979) analysis of rationalizing and covering errors in medical work reveals their utility in preserving the medical social fabric. Mechanic (1979a) describes the disinclination of physicians to control or sanction one another and debunks the myth that medical school is an effective screening process for ensuring quality and ethicality. He notes, however, that the myth has served the profession well in limiting external public scrutiny.

A final major proposal with regard to health organization relates to the issue of control within the system. From the perspective of those with chronic illness, control over as many decisions as possible ought to be afforded the chronically ill patient and family. However, the system dictates that most major decisions be made by someone "in authority," usually a physician or an officer of the bureaucratic structure (Freidson, 1981). This places patients and families in the unenviable position of having to learn the culture of health care delivery in order to develop ways of influencing its decision making on their behalf. From the perspective of patients and families, health care for chronic illness ought to be designed on the basis of assumptions other than those applicable in acute illness, that patients are passive and compliant recipients of the generosity of the experts. Analysts represented in the literature tend to agree (Schwartz, 1987). One woman's suggestion captures such a wistful desire to retain control over her own illness management. As she explained, "I would be my own health care professional. That's the ideal."

Thus, chronically ill patients and their families think that the health care system needs to take heed of the way in which it views patients. By treating them as "guinea pigs," by withholding information or being dishonest about their disease, and by assuming the right to make decisions on behalf of perfectly competent people, the health care system creates an intolerable climate for those with chronic illness. What it lacks, according to many of the patients and families in this study, is "respect":

> I basically believe, with everything, with all ages, from infants on, that there has to be an attitude of respect for one another. And whatever the age, I think that's the essential ingredient. Perhaps the medical person would respect me as a patient and I would respect them for whatever, and not just in the line of duty. Maybe that's where there's a failing sometimes, is that has to be an attitude to people in general.

However, according to Fox (1990), such respect is made almost impossible under conditions of medical education and health care work that are themselves brutalizing and dehumanizing.

From the accounts of chronically ill people and the writings of health care analysts, therefore, health care organization needs radical revision to meet the needs of the chronically ill. Bureaucratic regulation and standardization, for example, should be revised to allow for individual differences and respect the competent decision making of those who are familiar with their ongoing care. When multiple services or professionals are involved, a coordinating function is essential. It seems that primary care physicians are incapable of fulfilling this role, largely because remuneration schemes serve as a disincentive. If they were made accessible to patients and families on an ongoing basis, many believe that nurses could successfully fill this void. However, in order to do justice to a coordinating function, nurses ought to have more authority in accessing services and more advantageous professional working conditions. In addition, the chronically ill and the theorists agree that modification of reimbursement schemes to permit nontechnological solutions is of critical importance to chronic illness care. Finally, all of these proposals hinge on an attitudinal change that is badly needed. Until patients are respected as human beings with rights, and until the chronically ill are respected as distinct from those with episodic sickness, health care will continue to create havoc in the lives of those with chronic illness.

BIOMEDICAL IDEOLOGY

According to professional analysts as well as people who require ongoing involvement, an important step in improving health care for chronic illness consists of altering the degree to which biomedical ideology has been uncritically adopted in our society (O'Neill, 1986). Because it is the framework underlying not only medical care but also most policies in health care delivery, the biomedical view of illness has been influential in creating many of the health care problems confronting the chronically ill (Zola, 1981). Because the lay public as well as the health professions have traditionally accepted the biomedical view, regardless of whether they understood it or articulated it as such, a curative, disease-oriented system has flourished everywhere in the developed world (Navarro, 1989).

The chronically ill individuals and families in this study tell us that there is an unacceptable lack of concern within medical science for the psychosocial components of illness experience. Because health care is directed by a profession oriented toward the biological and pathophysiological implications of disease, the subjective state of health itself does not figure into most health services (Arney & Bergen, 1984; Fabrega, 1982). This mind-body distinction, in which subjective knowledge is considered idiosyncratic, irrational, and unreliable, derives from the Cartesian dualism underlying biomedical thought (Sullivan, 1986). As Gish (1984) points out, the essentially social character of our lives, which includes all of the problems associated with health and disease, is almost obliterated once we enter the health care system as patients. According to Rawlinson (1983), modern medicine fails to recognize the subjectivity of its subject in that it considers the human body as a mere corporeal entity, rather than as a living, intentional embodiment.

Patients and families also make it clear that the biomedical view fragments an understanding of illness into organ systems rather than meaningful components of the life experience. As other authors have noted, the lay public seems increasingly estranged from a view that reduces them to mere biological processes (Calnan & Williams, 1992; Kaufman, 1988). Because each medical specialty interprets the whole picture according to the unique dictates of its particular biological components, patients are given conflicting messages about their disease and its implications. Cockerham (1986) points out that the biomedical perspective leads practitioners to deal with chronic illness in much the same way that they formerly dealt with communicable diseases, although the conditions are fundamentally different. From the patient's and the family's point of view, therefore, much of what is considered medical service actually satisfies the curiosity of biomedical scientists rather than satisfying the quality of life concerns of those with ongoing illness.

The scientific basis of medicine is also called into question by chronically ill patients and families. Because they are the recipients of conflicting opinions, erroneous assumptions, and logical incongruities, many of those who live with chronic illness come to understand medical science as a form of argument rather than an objective window into the truth. As Armstrong (1987) explains, truth in medical science actually refers only to a momentary match with a classification system that is under constant revision. Further, according to Zaner (1983), the practice of medicine includes numerous regions of error. In ongoing situations such as chronic illness, medical truth rapidly changes. Thus, over time, their exposure to the frank subjectivity of diagnosis, labeling, prognosticating, and intervening leads those with chronic illness to reinterpret medical science as anything but logical. According to several theorists, the principle of specific causation, ingrained in biomedical logic, is responsible for the tunnel vision of medical science (Conrad & Schneider, 1981; McKeown, 1988; Mechanic, 1986a). As Travis (1980) explains, the notion that alleviating the specific cause of a disease will produce health is a gross oversimplification that continues to be perpetuated in medical science:

> The first step requires a letting go, in practice as well as in theory, of the archaic belief that disease is something which "happens" to us, at the direction of random forces "out there." I was taught in medical school that germs *cause* infections. I am now convinced that they are not the actual cause, but are only the mechanism by which I manifest the infection. The "bugs" are always around; but what caused me to lower my resistance and get the infection when the person next to me didn't? That question, if asked, would lead us to the real cause of the problem. (pp. 341-342)

Further, the role of professionals, especially physicians, derives from this biomedical understanding of what constitutes illness and wellness. As guardians of the mysteries of medical science, physicians and their allies have been well trained in conveying an attitude of certainty that their view is correct and confidence that their expertise surpasses that of all others involved (Freel, 1985; Freidson, 1986). This attitude is so deeply ingrained in medical practice that it creates the pattern of what has been described as "benevolent paternalism" underlying chronic illness care (Cohen, 1987).

This attitude also explains the historic and intense animosity of practitioners of "regular" medicine toward the universe of alternative health services (Brown, 1979; Conrad & Schneider, 1981; Worsley, 1982). As Baer (1989) notes, the approach of biomedicine to alternative medical systems can be characterized by the processes of annihilation, restriction, and absorption. Although they are generally discredited as unscientific, there is evidence that some of the beliefs inherent in these alternatives are shared by much of the population, including health care professionals themselves (Hepburn, 1988; Hillier, 1987; Roberson, 1987). As an indication of the extent to which nontraditional health care is entrenched in Western society, Halpern, Fisk, and Sobel (1984) estimate the size of the American health care counter-system at 3% of that nation's GNP. However, despite their increasing popularity, alternative treatment systems are marginal to the health care systems of all Western nations (Kleinman, 1984; Taylor, 1984). For chronically ill patients and their families, the animosity between regular medicine and its competitors prohibits rational collaboration:

> I think if everybody could just kind of . . . have a basic understanding of the practice of other professions, I think they could see that they're not being cut out by these other people, but they're just other supportive areas that each can support each other, and form a circle, you know, that would be able to completely take care of the whole person. . . . I guess that would be the best, you know, because then it seems like everybody would be using their abilities to the best.

Because the chronically ill, by the very nature of their affliction, must become competent in the everyday management of their illness, conflict between health care professionals and chronically ill patients seems inevitable. The accounts of patients and families reflect their difficulty overcoming the ingrained assumption that lay persons are incapable of making decisions with regard to their own health care. Indeed, it has been argued that members of Western society have been systematically indoctrinated toward deferring all health issues to doctors (Fox, 1986; Taylor, 1979; Zola, 1981). For example, Shorter (1985) cites a 1935 medical advertising campaign in which parents are admonished, in morbid and graphic terms, against self-diagnosing the common cold. Clearly, the message underlying that particular campaign was that untold miseries result from trying to take responsibility for even simple health decisions. In the aftermath of such social indoctrination during the medical profession's evolutionary phase, the overwhelming public willingness to relegate health decisions to doctors seems quite understandable (Taylor, 1979). Thus, from the patient perspective, the socially constructed medical role of expert in all health matters requires a radical revision in order to adapt to the needs of the chronically ill.

Biomedical ideology also emerges in the orientation of physicians and other health professionals toward curative services (Margolese, 1987). Because the human body is understood as a machine, the goal of medicine becomes fixing broken parts (Berliner, 1984; O'Neill, 1985). In the case of chronic illness, cures are not forthcoming. Thus, from the patient's and family's perspective, the health care system loses interest. Because status in professional medicine is derived from cures, especially dramatic ones, the chronically ill, with little hope for a cure, are relegated to the lowest status among patient populations (Hahn & Kleinman, 1983).

> Suffice it to say that the humdrum, the prosaic and the mundane have little place either in medical education or in much of the acquired self-understanding of health professionals. The prominence of combative, military, or warfare metaphors is clear enough, as are the various values they evoke: bravery, perseverance, valour in the face of overwhelming and implacable odds. (Zaner, 1984, p. 59)

Even among those who elect to practice their profession among the chronically ill, remnants of the champion mentality are apparent in the persistence of professionals in preserving authority over all aspects of illness management. Thus, the ideology sets up conditions in which chronically ill patients are forced to pretend to a subservient attitude while retaining control of their lives.

While chronically ill patients and families are not adverse to medical research toward a cure for their disease, many come to view the curative imperative as an exercise in academic medicine, advancing professional careers rather than generating a genuine source of information for the betterment of patients' lives. From their perspective, there are numerous aspects of illness care that beg immediate financial support, and pressing questions about quality of life that demand study. Due to the biomedical orientation to health, diverting economic resources to what would help patients is often impossible because they have been committed to the pursuit of a science which might someday provide answers (Black et al., 1986; Thomasma, 1984). One woman's desperation is evident in her analysis of this dilemma:

> I wish there was more funding for people like that. They need more, desperately, because the MS Society can do some great things, you know, by just talking, listening, understanding. . . . There has to be more funding for that sort of thing. They've cut it back so badly. It's all gone into research, you see. There's no money left over for patient services. . . . You know, some people are desperate for somebody to talk to. Desperate. And I'm one of them, I guess. I've been rambling on, for what—3 hours?

The impact of a cure orientation upon medical research funding has been well documented in the literature. According to Sanders (1985), certain potentially curable conditions are highly researched and highly resourced. Other more "class conscious" diseases, such as bronchitis, tend to be ignored. An obvious interpretation is that the most profitable sectors of the market are also the most appealing to medical researchers. Zaner further attributes current directions in medical research to its historical marriage to the natural sciences and the problems inherent in the Cartesian tradition:

> If nature, after all, is thought to be nothing but particles in motion and definable by mathematical formulas, then everything not so construable must be cast aside or into the "merely subjective." And so far as mathematical measurement became the paradigm of knowledge itself, anything not amenable to that mode of expression had to be regarded either as reducible to quantitative data (if it were to be knowable), or if not that, then taken as nonexistent or insignificant—that is, without efficacy and thus to be ignored as such. But this includes, after all, the entire range of values and thereby that of life. (1983, p. 143)

Dubious about the goals of medicine in society, Thomasma (1984) wonders what could possibly transform our steadily increasing tendency to ask only the small questions and treat only the definable problems.

From the perspective of those with chronic illness, the biomedical imperative clearly is not the ideal framework from which health care planning ought to be conducted. Burish and Bradley (1983) agree, and claim that application of the biomedical model toward problems in chronic illness is in part to blame for the current crisis in health care. Because it is so deeply ingrained in the public psyche, and so strongly entrenched in health care organization, biomedical ideology is understood to be a major roadblock to effecting meaningful changes in health care. As one patient points out, "It's a public image that needs to be changed."

The literature reveals ample evidence to confirm that the assumptions, categorization systems, and principles that underlie biomedical thought are thoroughly embedded in Western culture (Hahn & Kleinman, 1983; Lazarus & Pappas, 1986; van der Steen & Thung, 1988). As Mechanic and Aiken (1986) point out, for example, biomedicine and high technology have captured our collective imaginations and continue to give medical care its momentum and credibility. It also seems probable that the transmission of these ideologic messages in health care interactions is generally an unintentional process, dimly perceived by the participants involved (Waitzkin, 1984, 1986). The health care professions perpetuate "correct" structuring of consumers through codes of propriety in education, systems of problem recognition, and solutions featuring pathology and dysfunction (Romanucci-Ross, 1982). Thus, according to Waitzkin (1986), the non-critical nature of medical discourse encourages the maintenance of a system that is itself a serious source of distress for patients.

Although there have been numerous efforts to modify the highly analytical, logico-rational way of thinking that has come to characterize biomedical ideology, if not Western thought itself, such cognitions have proven highly resistant to change, both inside and outside the medical profession (Fox, 1990). However, there are some who foresee a revolution in the way Westerners understand the world. According to Pelletier (1980), paradigm shifts in science and the holistic health movement in medicine are evidence of this trend. What is clearly required in this regard is a major thrust in health care criticism toward unraveling the myth of biomedical superiority in health care planning for chronic illness.

From the perspectives of the lay critics and professional analysts presented here, it seems evident that biomedicine currently serves as a powerful social and cultural underpinning to the delivery of health care services for the chronically ill. What is badly needed in its place is a system that values people over machines, quality of life over cure, and competence over subservience. A thorough critical review is essential in professional education, in public awareness, and in the organization of health care delivery systems. Toward this end, health care consumers and policy analysts alike have urged public criticism of medical dominance and the biomedical imperative.

SOCIAL POLICY

A final theme in the analysis of the course ahead reflects an interpretation of health care as a matter of social policy. Underlying the changes required in both health care organization and biomedical ideology is the necessity to modify the policies that permit them to flourish. As was made evident in the accounts of chronically ill people and their families, distinctions between health and other aspects of social life are quite artificial. Well-being, from the perspective of the chronically ill, requires financial security, supportive social relations, productivity, and dignity. Where these are denied or inaccessible, health is inherently in jeopardy. This manufactured distinction between health and other sectors of society has been addressed by many health care analysts (Levine, Feldman, & Elinson, 1983; Mechanic, 1986a). They too argue that the position of health care organization within the social structure ought not dominate our interpretation of the health field to the exclusion of such equally significant factors as human biology, environment, and life-style (LaLonde, 1980; Siler-Wells, 1988).

Within the health sector, people with chronic illness report inequities that they deem detrimental to their ability to obtain the services necessary for an acceptable quality of life. First, they express frustration at major investments in hospital and institutional care at the expense of more economical services that would allow people to remain in the community:

> You know, this is the part that gets me. I can't understand why sometimes they'll leave you lying around in a bed and just leave you reading a book for days and days. You know, it doesn't take very many days when you're inactive that all your muscles just absolutely go to jelly and it doesn't take more than a week until you can hardly lift a cup of tea to your mouth.

That the system favors hospital care over less expensive options is well documented in the literature (Arney & Bergen, 1984). As Nield and Mahon (1981) explain, the preference for expensive forms of health care delivery is a consequence of the profit they represent to hospitals and health care providers: "More specifically, it is monetarily more advantageous for the health care system to maintain and promote crisis-generated care" (p. 27). Anderson (1990) agrees that the absence of effective home care support systems makes sense only in the context of a capitalist world system, in which the corporate elite has considerable input into health policy. It has clearly been recognized at a global level that making technical, hospital-based medicine available to the majority of the world's population is impossible (Worsley, 1982). Thus, Schwartz (1987) notes that, rather than social policy, the vested interests of stakeholders in the system determine how and where health care is delivered.

Where home support services exist, however, their exclusion criteria are seen as excessively rigid, reflecting a highly arbitrary definition of what constitutes appropriate service. As Walkover (1988) points out, in an era of cost containment, the first response of many social programs is to reduce the pool of potential beneficiaries by tightening eligibility restrictions. While they recognize that such regulation is probably the system's way of protecting itself against an onslaught of customers, should it expand its services too far from basic support for medical care, patients and families point out that such regulation leaves them no option but to manipulate the system. From their point of view, the costs of running a system in which people are constantly manipulative must be far higher than the costs of offering some of the basic services that people feel they need in order to maintain a reasonable quality of life with chronic illness. Further, they expect that there must be less restrictive and more creative ways in which necessary controls could be exerted. As one family proposes, "Well, it could be equalized through the tax system somehow, you know. You can equalize it by just getting it back from your taxes at the end of the year."

Second, the informants in this study note the absence of effective family support for coping with chronic illness in the home. One mother expresses the need for such support in the context of caring for chronically ill children at home:

> I think there's a serious lapse in the kind of attention that the health system, in particular in medicine, but the health system in general, can do for families that do have kids that have problems that can't be fixed.

From their perspective, the family serves as a significant source of health care for the chronically ill. However, formal recognition of that contribution and support for its maintenance is sadly lacking. This serious gap has also been acknowledged in the health care literature (Anderson, 1986; Meister, 1989; Woods, Yates, & Primomo, 1989).

Chronically ill people and their families further note that preventative and health promotion services, by far the most cost-effective option in their opinion, receive an insignificant proportion of all health care funding. For those with chronic illness, access to the resources necessary to prevent acute episodes and to maintain the best possible level of wellness seem logical, from both a humane and a financial perspective. One man's description of his extended physiotherapy illustrates this view:

> I'm sure that if I hadn't done some of these things, that I would've been a burden for years and years and years and years. So, to me, really getting that quality time, and focusing, and communicating, and doing the right kind of work is worth the time, even money-wise, even though in the short run it doesn't look that way, 'cause it costs a lot of money.

In essence, these patients and families see the current patterns of resource allocation as locking the barn door after the horse has fled. This dismal view of the traditional approach to chronic illness care is shared by many health care analysts (Butterfield, 1990; Warr, 1981). However, because prevention is scarcely apparent in most medical school curricula (Cockerham, 1986), medicine is hardly likely to lead the way in the direction of preventative care. Thus, one important social policy shift required for effective health care system reform involves widening the extremely narrow vision of health that characterizes the existing health sector (Harris, 1989; Vojtecky, 1986).

Another area in which those with chronic illness notice incongruity is the salary differential between various health care workers. In their view, certain workers, such as medical specialists, are able to command excessive salaries in relation to the benefit they give patients. Others, such as hospital nurses and paraprofessionals, are grossly underpaid for the obvious effort they expend on the patients' behalf:

> I also think that what it would take would be like health care professionals who were getting a decent wage for perhaps working less hours, so that they're not under a lot of stress. So that they could be on, and productive, when they're doing their work. Because I think that people are only human, and working in bad working conditions at low wages for long hours is not

very good for health care people. People then, they get burned out, and they can't give their best.

It seems that consumers in the health care system support decent remuneration as long as it demonstrably benefits the health of patients. As one of the study's informants points out, "It goes right back to where our values as a culture lie."

In the current scholarly literature, there is considerable evidence that a similar argument is being posed by health care analysts and economists. While the tradition in Western countries has been to allow medicine substantial input into health policy and resource allocation, it has been argued that there is no basis in biomedicine for considering the larger social benefit of various health care decisions (Illich, 1975; Last, 1988; Mechanic, 1986a). Because biomedicine's target is exclusively the individual, success is typically measured in the context of individual gains rather than any collective benefits (Levine et al., 1983). Further, it is generally understood that the consuming public demands this to be so (Halpern et al., 1984).

The accounts of the chronically ill patients and families in this study suggest that, at least in the case of chronic illness, health care consumers are capable of a surprisingly sophisticated analysis of the larger picture in health care. In contrast, health care planning has often resembled clinical decision making more than it has social analysis (Drummond, 1987). Interpretations of the health of societies, by physicians as well as many other health care analysts, have tended to reflect biomedical definitions. The conventional indicators typically used to evaluate the health of nations are more likely to include information about the number of physicians and hospital beds per capita than actual measures of health status within the population (Sanders, 1985).

Complicating the matter is a death-denying Western culture in which preservation of human life is the highest standard against which to evaluate the cost-benefit ratio of any medical intervention. Whether the cost of any lifesaving measure is justifiable in terms of the health of the society as a whole is beyond the scope of biomedical theory (Daniels, 1985). Failing to recognize that limitation, proponents of biomedicine continue to bankrupt society to "save" individual lives without having to account for the larger destructive implications that such policies inevitably create (Besharov & Silver, 1989; Simmons & Marine, 1984).

Further, as Sanders (1985) indicates, most of the world's population lives in rural areas, and most of the spending on medical care is in urban areas, where most doctors and other health care workers reside. Moreover, three-quarters of the deaths are due to conditions that can be prevented at low cost, while three-quarters of the medical budget is spent on curative services, many of them at high cost. Indeed, maldistribution is reported to be a significant problem in the health care systems of all capitalist countries (Light, 1986; Starr, 1981; Waitzkin, 1983b). Thus, because they are seen as the domain of other sectors, such escalating social problems as homelessness, infant mortality, drug addiction, and alienation are not figured into the accounting of how health resources ought to be distributed within a society (Taylor, 1979).

As Schilling (1981) notes, although the ethical dilemmas raised by acute illness have attracted more attention, those inherent in chronic illness care are no less significant. Increasingly, chronic illness is overrepresented in two population groups with little political clout, the aged and the poor (Funkhouser & Moser, 1990). Such trends will increasingly confront policymakers with the necessity of facing difficult questions about the morality of allowing costly health care decisions to be made at individual levels while entire populations are suffering.

According to Sanders (1985), we tend to assume that illness ought to be resolved at the individual level, even when its causes are thought to be social in origin. In this way, medicine serves the interests of those in power and preserves the existing social order. However, as Waitzkin (1984) points out, illnesses associated with social problems require resistance, activism, and political organizing. These questions of cost-effectiveness, evaluation, and ethics all demand some sort of moral evaluation within society with regard to how it ought to treat its members. Is professional autonomy worth the price of escalated suffering? What is the social value of any given human life? How long can the interests of individuals be protected if the rights of the collective are threatened? And who will ultimately decide? Such questions will increasingly demand answers, not only in theory but also in social policy.

Remuneration schemes are another important element in the social policy of health care for chronic illness. Canadian chronically ill patients and their families appreciate that they do have access to resources whose cost might be prohibitive in countries without an adequate health insurance scheme. However, they also have serious concerns about the implications of health service reimbursement under the existing system. As has been noted, they believe that current fee-for-service billing regulations often overload the system rather than control its use effectively. Further, they notice that these same regulations seem to bias decision making toward obtaining the most expensive alternatives, such as hospitalization, unnecessary diagnostic procedures, and specialty consultation. As an illustration, they contrast the frequency with which physicians refer them to psychiatrists to deal with their emotional distress to the intense resistance of those same physicians to patient support groups. From their point of view, the lack of financial incentives to provide patients with the most economical and logical service delivery options creates a climate in which professionals take little responsibility for their excesses. At the same time, spokespersons for the medical profession, in explanation of accelerating health care costs, often blame patients for overextending the system (Dean, 1986; Salmon, 1984).

The lay and scholarly analyses also point out that remuneration schemes and profit motives influence health care significantly, even in a highly regulated system (Griffith, Iliffe, & Rayner, 1987; Marmor & Dunham, 1983; Susser, Hopper, & Richman, 1983). They suggest that the myth of the altruistic health care professional ought to be given proper burial, and the self-interest of the professions openly challenged (Fox, 1986; Taylor, 1979). As Sanders (1985) points out, those in private medical practice in developed countries will generally serve in the localities that can best afford them. Swartz (1977) further notes that in systems with greater public regulation, those who benefit the most are the professions, not the patients. As a result, self-interest is evident, regardless of the remuneration pattern.

The arguments on how remuneration policies actually influence health care are intense and heated in the scholarly literature. For example, because Canada and the United States hold similar ethics of professional autonomy but different rules regarding how services will be remunerated, the two are often compared for insights on how remuneration enacts social policy (Sullivan, 1990). Kaufmann (1987) characterizes the essential policy distinction as one of defining health care as a right (Canada) or a commodity (the United States). However, in both nations, the traditional resistance of physicians to nationalized health insurance schemes has been intense (Kaufmann, 1987; Marmor & Dunham, 1983). In addition, both have been able to maintain a remuneration structure that relies heavily upon fee-for-service.

Although the medical profession typically argues that fee-for-service is an essential requisite for autonomous professional practice, there are many who feel that it specifically influences service delivery and even clinical decisions in chronic illness care, since the services needed by the chronically ill are notoriously low on the remuneration scale. While the tendency with fee-for-service is that the most lucrative services become the most popular, prepaid schemes can create different sorts of dilemmas for chronic illness care, according to some theorists (Crum, 1991). As Schlesinger (1986) argues, instead of biasing clinical decisions toward what is most immediately lucrative, such schemes tend to bias decisions toward what is most cost-effective for the plan. In both cases, then, the chronically ill may be the hardest hit, since actually quantifying the cost-effectiveness of preventative and health promotion activities in chronic care is often impossible.

Accordingly, the chronically ill and the health care analysts agree that how professionals are remunerated influences the service that they will provide. Because the requirements of the chronically ill are radically different from those with episodic illness, however, it seems probable that remuneration schemes in chronic illness care ought not to borrow models designed in relation to other types of health care. Social policy in this regard, therefore, demands that the special requirements of various forms of health care be analyzed differently, perhaps requiring a variety of remuneration schemes within a single health care system.

A related economic issue of great concern to chronically ill patients and families is the fact that certain sectors of society make a profit from health care. While the profit motive may be less visible in a system that is nationally insured, its influence is felt nonetheless. Those living with chronic illness point to the pharmaceutical and medical supplies industries as being directly invested in retaining a market for their products, rather than promoting well-being. As a population whose needs are ongoing, the chronically ill feel particularly vulnerable to such market manipulations in health care.

In addition to their chagrin about the profit motive of the health industries, chronically ill patients and their families have grave concerns about the degree to which health care professionals themselves stand to profit from the various clinical decisions they make. They recognize that relations between these professions and the health industries are cozy, and suspect there are many in the health care and the private sector whose livelihood rests on their remaining ill. As Spicker (1988) points out, it is difficult for the public to view physicians as "disinterested trustees" in social planning roles if those same individuals are stakeholders in the business of investing in the misfortune of others.

While the entrepreneurial role of physicians in Canada is clearly more restricted than it seems to be south of the border (Relman, 1987), there is no doubt that financial incentives within all capitalist societies make the health care industry a lucrative investment (Caplan, 1989; de Swaan, 1989). According to Waitzkin (1983a), there is no mechanism within free enterprise to prevent the exploitation of illness for private profit. Further, there is little possibility of restraining the private sector from influencing social policy regarding health care if there is a profit to be had (Altman, 1986). Even more horrifying is the idea that there are larger profits to be made in manufacturing illness than in curing it (McKinlay, 1981a). Thus, while patients and their families may focus on specific industries as being particularly invested in their ill health, it seems that the problem may be even more pervasive and insidious.

Consideration of the arguments in favor of multisectoral policy, accountability for resource allocation, remuneration schemes appropriate to chronic illness, and restrictions on the profit potential reflects the adamant position, of both consumers and health care analysts, that the problems in health care ought to be considered within the larger context of general social policy. For those with chronic illness, the resources necessary for health include those within the domains of many sectors, but are controlled by the definitional frameworks of a single orientation to health and illness. Because policy is often enacted within and not between sectors, coordinated chronic illness care is next to impossible. Thus, health reform for chronic illness clearly requires structural revision within governing bodies at both local and national levels (Milio, 1988).

In Western capitalist societies, health care models based on competitive incentives are often considered essential motivators in improving health care (Ben-Sira, 1988; Rogers & Barnard, 1979). Analysts who refrain from criticism of the dominant mode of production are therefore restricted to reform proposals that consider ways of humanizing the existing system by creating financial incentives for their proposed changes (de Vries, Berg, & Lipkin, 1982). In contrast, as has been apparent in the discussion thus far, many health care analysts believe that capitalism itself actually poses one of the most serious threats to health care reform (McKinlay & Stoeckle, 1988). As Swartz (1977) explains, no capitalist society is capable of effecting policies that place collective consumption above personal consumption, or human development over economic development. The accounts of patients suggest that such policies are indeed what would be needed for effective reform of health care for chronic illness. However, the extent to which the expressed interests of the public can influence health policy at the social level within capitalism is questionable (Navarro, 1984).

Capitalism further produces inherent resistance to such policy reforms as equitable resource allocation, local community involvement, and the emphasis on preventative health (Baer, Singer, & Johnsen, 1986). Because of its tendency to reproduce structures of class relations, capitalism also permits those invested in technological biomedical care systems to maintain and enhance their grasp over policy within the health care system (Tomes, 1985). As Sanders (1985) adds, medicine's investment in the developing world, for example, has served to reinforce political and economic systems that are the direct cause of ill health. Thus, as many have argued, it seems likely that the concern for capital accumulation, in combination with the profit promotion of the medical industry, is at the root of many of the problems in health care today (McKee, 1988).

Among critical theorists, there are many who see hope for the future in socializing the health care industry. As Waitzkin (1983a) argues, cost containment cannot occur without compulsory restriction of health care profit and the eventual public ownership of medical industries. From his vantage point, true reform in health care is impossible without social and political revolution (1983b). Pointing to the success of Cuba and some other socialist countries in advancing preventative medicine, Worsley (1982) explains that reform which does not change the monopoly of biomedicine, the professional autonomy of physicians, and the involvements of corporate interests will have little effect on the system overall.

By transplanting the discussion of health care reform into the theater of massive social and political reform, the complexity of the problem in modern health care is made evident. Clearly, there are no obvious solutions. Even when the overall goals are remarkably similar, there is extreme diversity of opinion on how to reach them (Mechanic, 1979a). In concert with the movement toward understanding health reform as social reform, however, there are many who locate hope for the future in the critical mass of people whose interpretation of health care has extended far beyond self-interest. According to many analysts, the existence of a self-care movement, a voluntary collaborative effort between people who have recognized problems inherent in the traditional way of understanding health care, may be the key to forging significant health care reform in the future (Ferguson, 1980; Hunt,

1988; Sanders, 1985). The ingredient underlying the success of this movement is its ability to free health care consumers from the bonds of individuality, and to confront them with their collective strength (Labonte, 1987). Critical change agents within the health sector of many Western nations are now beginning to develop increasingly imaginative methods for drawing out this collective potential within local communities and fostering its influence over public policy (Hancock, 1987; Watts, 1990).

Such a trend is consistent with what the World Health Organization has advocated for global health reform (Law & Lariviere, 1988). As Milio (1988) points out, short of radical social revolution, the use of broad public policy to effect major changes in health care organization, delivery, and definition is the only available option. The concept of "healthy public policy" is beginning to appear in the literature as an orientation toward evaluating all social policy on the basis of its explicit concern for health and equity, as well as its accountability for health impact (Callahan, 1992; O'Neill, 1989/90).

To effect change, however, this new critical mass movement will have to overcome the internalized values of the majority with regard to the role of biomedicine in health care. Because a social movement such as this has little access to the means by which such values are socialized, and no capacity to change the institutional reward infrastructures (Turner, 1986), ideological shifts in health care will obviously be painful and protracted. And because biomedical ideology is so ingrained in our Western culture, a willingness for intense collective introspection will therefore be indispensable to the forces of change.

More optimistically, the growing strength of the health care consumer movement and the increasingly vocal criticism by health care analysts may be interpreted as hopeful signs of a paradigm shift in progress. That chronically ill people discern the same issues and logical flaws as do scholarly health care critics speaks to the validity of the collective interpretations. As MacGregor (1974) argued some time ago, the steps toward solutions in health care are contained within the ingredients of Western thought itself. From his point of view, a new orientation could form the basis of the eventual solutions. He recognized a life-centered philosophy over the aggrandizement of the human species, collectivism over individualism, naturalism over rationalism, meaning over materialism, and change over growth as essential shifts in the way we view ourselves and our universe. As we know, such arguments have been put forward by many critics of Western thinking, and have become comfortable for an increasing number of thoughtful minds.

The stories of the chronically ill have enlightened us about the meaning of having ongoing illness in our society. They have horrified us with the distress that a troubled health care system can inflict on such a vulnerable segment of the population. Further, they have convinced us that something is terribly wrong in health care, and that a rather radical reform is urgently required.

However, health care reform is not a problem distinct from all the others that currently face us as we look toward the end of a century of unprecedented "progress." Perhaps, as health care analysts, environmentalists, human rights activists, and all manner of dissatisfied people learn to appreciate the commonalities within their struggles, a meaningful social change can be envisioned. As we strive to ask questions outside our own universe of concern, as we look to the leadership of social critics of all orientations, and as we learn to respect the value of the struggle itself, perhaps we can begin to make the necessary cognitive links to see ourselves as part of a global community in evolution.

Appendix—Methodological Issues

BACKGROUND: THE CURRENT RESEARCH

The research that forms the basis for this book attempts to answer the very general question: How do patients and their families experience chronic illness? Drawing upon the naturalistic approach of Lincoln and Guba (1985) as a foundation for design and process decisions, it reflects primary and secondary analysis of data gathered over the course of several qualitative studies, each of which addressed some aspect of chronic illness experience. Previous research by this author in the area of cancer experience (Thorne, 1985, 1986, 1988) had initiated a fascination for the degree to which subjective illness experience was shaped by encounters in health care. In collaboration with Carole Robinson, whose own research into the experience of parents of chronically ill children had produced similar conclusions, a secondary analysis of our combined data sets, using grounded theory as our reference (Glaser & Strauss, 1967), generated a tentative theory about the evolution of trust in ongoing health care relationships (Robinson & Thorne, 1985; Thorne & Robinson, 1988a).

On the basis of this tentative theory, we mounted a grounded theory study of health care relationships in chronic illness, interviewing more than 70 people experienced in health care relationships for a chronic illness over a 3-year period. Constant comparative analysis of the evolving data set, using a research team, allowed us to confirm the strength of our original conceptualization of the stages through which health care relationships evolve, as well as to generate a typology of relationship types that emerge within the resolution phase (Thorne & Robinson, 1989).

In subsequent collaborative work, I began to explore the possibilities of tapping the existing database for the purpose of answering new, but related, research questions. In this context, I conducted additional studies on the experience of the subset of chronically ill mothers (Thorne, 1990b) and on the phenomenon of noncompliance in chronic illness (Thorne, 1990a). These inquiries convinced me of the tremendous value of the extensive existing database and gave me confidence to embark on the larger project that is the subject of this book.

The current project therefore capitalized on the existence of this large, rich, and extensive database consisting of accounts of health care relationships in chronic illness (summarized in Chapters 5 and 6). Because explaining such a phenomenon necessitates contextualizing the health care relationship within a particular illness experience, people tended to tell their stories from the beginning, and thus the original interviews included considerable material that was used only incidentally in the health care relationships work. Further, the accounts pointed to a much larger issue, in that the informants expressed their unique experiences in the context of a macro interpretation of issues and problems within the health care system as a whole. While their analysis of social organization of health care went far beyond the scope of that original project, I was sufficiently intrigued to pursue it further.

SECONDARY ANALYSIS

Secondary analysis is the process of using existing data sources for purposes other than that for which they were originally created (Woods, 1988). While it is highly dependent on the nature and quality of the original data sources, its advantages include both efficient use of existing material and capitalizing on broader population samples than one would otherwise be able to obtain. Because it requires that the researcher accept the database as it exists, without recourse to redesigning the study, the "fit" between the data and the research question is critical in determining whether secondary analysis will serve the researcher's purposes (McArt & McDougal, 1985).

In this instance, having been immersed in the original data construction, I was quite familiar with the database's scope and extent. Further, the fit between the research question and the existing data set was excellent. However, because my secondary analysis questions were not the intended focus of the original research, I acknowledged that there would be some variability in the extent to which individual informants addressed each of the larger themes. Drawing upon the "emergent design" principle in naturalistic inquiry (Lincoln & Guba, 1985), I therefore used the database as a beginning, and conducted additional focused interviews with new informants throughout the study to clarify and validate my interpretations. Such a design plan enabled me to obtain optimal advantage from the existing source without limiting me to its original scope.

DATA COLLECTION

A brief overview of processes used to construct the database will explain the range and depth of data that was generated in the primary studies as well as the later interviews. Volunteer participation was recruited through advertisements in newsletters of various disease-related advocacy organizations; presentations to self-help groups; and notices posted in clinics. Some informants were referred directly by colleagues or friends; others self-referred after hearing from a friend or support group peer about the interview experience.

Recruitment focused on participants who had ongoing physical illnesses. Although people with primary psychological or cognitive illnesses, and those who were imminently terminal, were specifically not recruited on the assumption that these conditions might represent distinct illness experiences, several of the informants did require psychological treatment or confront life-threatening illness during the project period. All the informants, then, had experience with a diagnosed chronic disease (in their own body or in that of a close family member) for which they had sought professional health care over time. More than half of the total of 91 informants had lived with chronic illness for longer than 10 years.

The recruitment strategy allowed for theoretical representation of a number of common and less common chronic diseases and conditions (see Table A.1). As it happened, several informants were simultaneously coping with multiple chronic conditions, either in the same patient or within the immediate family. In order to represent the family as well as the patient perspective in the analysis, parents of chronically ill children as well as people intimately involved in health care for chronically ill adult family members were recruited (see Table A.2). The gender distribution of informants was typical of patterns identified by other researchers using volunteer subjects. Although the ages of informants ranged from preteens to individuals in their nineties, the majority of informants were middle adults.

TABLE A.1 Chronic Illnesses Represented in the Study Population
(Total informants = 91; Total illnesses = 107)

Respiratory disease	14	Dermatological problems	3
Cardiovascular disease	13	Cystic Fibrosis	2
Arthritis	13	Hypertension	2
Chronic back/neck pain	13	Thyroid dysfunction	2
Inflammatory Bowel Disease	10	Epilepsy	2
Multiple Sclerosis	7	Chronic pancreatitis	1
Orthopedic problems	7	Myasthenia Gravis	1
Scleroderma	4	Endometriosis	1
Diabetes	4	Cerebral Palsy	1
Phenylketonuria	3	Renal disease	1
Gastric ulcer	3	Anemia	1

TABLE A.2 Sample Characteristics ($N = 91$)

Chronically ill individuals	60 (65.9%)
Family members	31 (34.1%)
Family of adult patients	18 (58.1%)
Parents of chronically ill children	13 (41.9%)
Female	59 (64.8%)
Male	32 (32.5%)

Ethical concerns were addressed by conforming to the requirements of the University of British Columbia's Screening Committee for Research Involving the Use of Human Subjects, from whom prior approval was obtained for both the primary and secondary studies. All informants were free to refuse to answer any questions or withdraw from the study at any time, and were assured that confidentiality and anonymity would be preserved.

One to four interviews with each informant took place in the home of the informant or in some other mutually agreeable location. Initial interviews were loosely guided by general questions intended to orient the account toward health care involvement. As the interviews progressed, specific questions emerging from the data were incorporated into the schedule for subsequent interviews to allow for clarification, validation, and expansion. All interviews were recorded on audiotape and later transcribed verbatim.

DATA ANALYSIS

Analysis of the emerging data occurred simultaneously with data collection. For the duration of the primary project, a research team met regularly to interpret transcripts and discuss emerging themes and categories. As categories within the data began to emerge, purposive sampling refined the additional recruitment, allowing a focus on specific aspects of the emerging theory. In the final phases, informants who had contributed to the conceptualization were asked to consider the conclusions prior to the preparation of the formal report. This process permitted confidence that the analytic framework held true for the informants and offered a useful interpretation of their experience.

The original database constructed for the Health Care Relationships Project included the accounts of 77 informants with firsthand experience in ongoing health care relationships for chronic illness. Following that project, and in relation to the evolving secondary research questions, an additional 14 informants were recruited and interviewed in a similar manner. All procedural and ethical practices were identical with those used in the primary study. However, as the focus of the research narrowed from the health care dyad to the larger health care system, the interviews focused more specifically on that phenomenon. In general, these secondary interviews augmented the existing database at the same time as they informed the emerging analysis, which became this study's conceptual framework.

The secondary analysis therefore relied on the data from both primary and secondary data constructions. It was guided by two research questions: How do chronically ill people and their families experience health care? and, How do chronically ill people and their families make sense of their experiences with health care? In its approach, the secondary application took general direction from the notion of explanatory models of illness experience (Kleinman, 1980; Kleinman et al., 1978). This model's claim, that inherent discrepancies in underlying belief systems between patients and practitioners shape the way in which illness is experienced, interpreted, and given meaning in our culture, makes explicit the rationale for eliciting the patient and family's perspective.

The secondary analysis was specifically informed by themes arising out of the primary analysis. While certain of these themes (such as the diagnosis story, the meaning of acute episodes, and the impact of visibility) had been acknowledged in memos made in the course of the primary study, none had been thoroughly analyzed in the primary application. In addition, new questions were posed regarding the way people interpret the experiences they have in searching for and obtaining help, and the way they understand the professional explanatory model underlying health care delivery. Because the informants sharing their illness narratives in the primary study also expressed the need to make sense of them in the larger scheme of things, the central questions of this secondary study were directly emergent from the earlier research.

Exploration of these questions allowed for the generation of an analytic framework from which all of these issues could be interpreted. From the perspective of the informants, chronic illness experience could be conceptualized as having distinct meanings at four levels of awareness: the biological level (in the sense of disease process or symptoms); the individual level (in the sense of one's unique subjective experience with illness); the social level (in terms of the interpersonal environment, including health care relationships, that shapes the experience with illness); and the structural level (the institutions and philosophies within which care for the illness must be negotiated). According to this framework, in order to appreciate any one level, the others must be addressed. Thus, the experience of chronic illness is understood as a complex and multidimensional whole in which all aspects are best understood in the context of the others.

The form in which this report is articulated reflects one way in which the "trustworthiness" of the findings is addressed (Catanzaro, 1988). Major themes are presented in such a way that they reflect a composite of informants' perspectives about each phenomenon, as well as the emergence of the researcher's analysis of the meaning inherent in the accounts. In keeping with the tradition that values "thick description" (Scheff, 1986), liberal use is made of verbatim quotations and anecdotes from individual informants. Each such reference is made by virtue not of its uniqueness but of some element that represents the shared experience. Thus, the writing style aims to create a portrait of the whole rather than a record of specific unique individuals. The reader will therefore come away with the sense of understanding the plot better than the individual characters in the play.

Since the central issue involved is one of human experience, this presentation style taps the range and variation in events, perspectives, and philosophies within the informant population to maximize the reader's own human connection with an informant's experience. The intent of the writing form is, therefore, to promote credibility, within the mind of the reader, for the analysis that is developed in the course of the description (Catanzaro, 1988) and auditability for the process through which it was derived (Sandelowski, 1986).

The mechanical aspects of analysis were managed through the use of established and adapted procedures. Immersion in the data, through transcript analysis and ongoing interviewing, generated the specific questions that directed this secondary analysis. Open and axial coding (Strauss & Corbin, 1990) of themes arising from this process created a set of notes reflecting ongoing conceptual formulation. When no new general themes were forthcoming, more formal analytic procedures were adopted. All data were converted into a word-processing format. Because of the sheer volume of data (which totalled 6,000 pages of verbatim transcript), I abandoned attempts to apply available software programs designed for qualitative data management, and instead used manually embedded codes and subsequent macro procedures to code and sort the data. Subsequently, inductive analysis of each theme was performed (Knafl & Webster, 1988). This additional step allowed for recoding and reorganization of ideas within each theme and in relation to the whole. It further provided a basis for judgment about the necessity for further inquiry, directed either to the data set or to additional informants. The final organizational structure of this book, therefore, reflects the fruits of this analytic process.

References

Alexander, L. (1982). Illness maintenance and the new American sick role. In N. J. Chrisman & T. W. Maretzki (Eds.), *Clinically applied anthropology: Anthropologists in health science settings* (pp. 351-367). Boston: D. Reidel.

Alonzo, A. A. (1984). An illness behavior paradigm: A conceptual exploration of a situational-adaptation perspective. *Social Science & Medicine, 19*, 499-510.

Alonzo, A. A. (1985). An analytical typology of disclaimers, excuses and justifications surrounding illness: A situational approach to health and illness. *Social Science & Medicine, 21*, 153-162.

Altman, D. E. (1986). Two views of a changing health care system. In L. H. Aiken & D. Mechanic (Eds.), *Applications of social science to clinical medicine and health policy* (pp. 100-112). New Brunswick, NJ: Rutgers University Press.

Amundsen, D. W., & Ferngren, G. B. (1983). Evolution of the patient-physician relationship: Antiquity through the Renaissance. In E. E. Shelp (Ed.), *The clinical encounter: The moral fabric of the patient-physician relationship* (pp. 3-46). Dordrecht, Holland: D. Reidel.

Anderson, J. M. (1986). Ethnicity and illness experience: Ideological structures and the health care delivery system. *Social Science & Medicine, 22*, 1277-1283.

Anderson, J. M. (1990). Home care management in chronic illness and the self-care movement: An analysis of ideologies and economic processes influencing policy decision. *Advances in Nursing Science, 12*(2), 71-83.

Anderson, W. T., & Helm, D. T. (1979). The physician-patient encounter: A process of reality negotiation. In E. G. Jaco (Ed.), *Patients, physicians, and illness* (pp. 259-271). New York: Free Press.

Appelbaum, P. S., & Roth, L. H. (1983). Patients who refuse treatment in medical hospitals. *Journal of the American Medical Association, 250*(10), 1296-1301.

Armstrong, D. (1983). *An outline of sociology as applied to medicine* (2nd ed.). Bristol, UK: Wright.

Armstrong, D. (1984). The patient's view. *Social Science & Medicine, 18*, 737-744.

Armstrong, D. (1987). Bodies of knowledge: Foucault and the problem of human anatomy. In G. Scambler (Ed.), *Sociological theory and medical sociology* (pp. 59-76). London: Tavistock.

Arney, W. R., & Bergen, B. J. (1984). *Medicine and the management of living: Taming the last great beast.* Chicago: University of Chicago Press.

Arpin, K., Fitch, M., Browne, G. B., & Corey, P. (1988). *The effectiveness and efficiency of family clinical appointments in promoting adjustment to chronic illness: An overview.* Unpublished manuscript, Ontario Minstry of Health, Toronto.

Baer, H. A. (1989) The American dominative medical system as a reflection of social relations in the larger society. *Social Science & Medicine, 28,* 1103-1112.

Baer, H. A., Singer, M., & Johnsen, J. H. (1986). Toward a critical medical anthropology. *Social Science & Medicine, 23,* 95-98.

Barnard, D. (1988). "Ship? What ship? I thought I was going to the doctor!": Patient-centered perspectives on the health care team. In N.M.P. King, L. R. Churchill, & A. W. Cross (Eds.), *The physician as captain of the ship: A critical appraisal* (pp. 89-111). Dordrecht, Holland: D. Reidel.

Baron, D. A. (1987). Emotional aspects of chronic disease. *Journal of the American Osteopathic Society, 87,* 437-439.

Becker, M. H. (1974). The health belief model and sick role behavior. *Health Education Monographs, 2,* 409-419.

Becker, M. H., Haefner, D. P., Kasl, S. V., Kirscht, J. P., Maiman, L. A., & Rosenstock, I. M. (1977). Selected psychosocial models and correlates of individual health-related behaviors. *Medical Care, 15*(5), 27-46.

Bennett, J. W. (1985). The micro-macro nexus: Typology, process, and system. In B. R. DeWalt & P. J. Pelto (Eds.), *Micro and macro levels of analysis in anthropology: Issues in theory and research* (pp. 23-54). Boulder, CO: Westview.

Ben-Sira, Z. (1984). Chronic illness, stress and coping. *Social Science & Medicine, 18*(9), 725- 736.

Ben-Sira, Z. (1988). *Politics and primary medical care: Dehumanization and overutilization.* Brookfield, VT: Avebury.

Berliner, H. S. (1984). Scientific medicine since Flexner. In J. W. Salmon (Ed.), *Alternative medicines: Popular and policy perspectives* (pp. 30-56). New York: Tavistock.

Besharov, D. J., & Silver, J. D. (1989). Rationing access to advanced medical techniques. In K. McLennan & J. A. Meyer (Eds.), *Care and cost: Current issues in health policy* (pp. 41-66). Boulder, CO: Westview.

Black, R. B., Dornan, D. H., & Allegrante, J. P. (1986). Challenges in developing health promotion services for the chronically ill. *Social Work, 31,* 287-293.

Bochner, S. (1983). Doctors, patients and their cultures. In D. Pendleton & J. Hasler (Eds.), *Doctor-patient communication* (pp. 127-138). London: Academic Press.

Bosk, C. L. (1979). *Forgive and remember: Managing medical failure.* Chicago: University of Chicago Press.

Bourhis, R. Y., Roth, S., & MacQueen, G. (1989). Communication in the hospital setting: A survey of medical and everyday language use amongst patients, nurses and doctors. *Social Science & Medicine, 28,* 339-346.

Brody, H. (1987). *Stories of sickness.* New Haven: Yale University Press.

Brown, M. C. (1979). The health care crisis in historical perspective. *Canadian Journal of Public Health, 79,* 300-306.

Buchanan, J. H. (1989). *Patient encounters: The experience of disease.* Charlottesville: The University Press of Virginia.

Buller, M. K., & Buller, D. (1987). Physicians' communication style and patient satisfaction. *Journal of Health & Social Behavior, 28,* 375-388.

Burish, T. G., & Bradley, L. A. (1983). Coping with chronic disease: Definitions and issues. In T. G. Burish & L. A. Bradley (Eds.), *Coping with chronic disease: Research and applications* (pp. 3-12). New York: Academic Press.

Bury, M. (1991). The sociology of chronic illness: A review of research and prospects. *Sociology of Health & Illness, 13*, 451-468.

Butterfield, P. G. (1990). Thinking upstream: Nurturing a conceptual understanding of the societal context of health behavior. *Advances in Nursing Science, 12*(2), 1-8.

Califano, J. A. (1986). *America's health care revolution: Who lives? Who dies? Who pays?* New York: Random House.

Callahan, D. (1992). Organizing a health care vision. In R. H. Blank & A. L. Bonnicksen (Eds.), *Emerging issues in biomedical policy: An annual review* (vol. 1, pp. 146-157). New York: Columbia University Press.

Calnan, M. (1984). Clinical uncertainty: Is it a problem in the doctor-patient relationship? *Sociology of Health & Illness, 6*(1), 74-85.

Calnan, M. (1987). *Health and illness: The lay perspective.* London: Tavistock.

Calnan, M., & Williams, S. (1992). Images of scientific medicine. *Sociology of Health & Illness, 14*, 233-254.

Cameron, P., Titus, D. G., Kostin, J., & Kostin, M. (1973). The life satisfaction of nonnormal persons. *Journal of Consulting and Clinical Psychology, 41*, 207-214.

Carlson, R. J. (1975). *The end of medicine.* New York: John Wiley.

Caplan, R. L. (1989). The commodification of American health care. *Social Science & Medicine, 28*, 1139-1148.

Catanzaro, M. (1988). Using qualitative analytic techniques. In N. F. Woods & M. Catanzaro, *Nursing research: Theory and practice* (pp. 437-456). St. Louis: Mosby.

Charmaz, K. (1983). Loss of self: A fundamental form of suffering in the chronically ill. *Sociology of Health and Illness, 5*, 168-197.

Chrisman, N. J., & Kleinman, A. (1983). Popular health care, social networks, and cultural meanings: The orientation of medical anthropology. In D. Mechanic (Ed.), *Handbook of health, health care, and the health professions* (pp. 569-590). New York: Free Press.

Cockerham, W. C. (1986). Health policy in selected industrial countries. In *Medical sociology* (3rd ed., pp. 246-266). Englewood Cliffs, NJ: Prentice-Hall.

Cohen, C. B. (1987). Patient autonomy in chronic illness. *Family and Community Health, 10*(1), 24-34.

Cohen, F., & Lazarus, R. S. (1983). Coping and adaptation in health and illness. In D. Mechanic (Ed.), *Handbook of health, health care, and the health professions* (pp. 608-635). New York: Free Press.

Cole, S., & Lejeune, R. (1987). Illness and the legitimation of failure. In H. D. Schwartz (Ed.), *Dominant issues in medical sociology* (2nd ed., pp. 31-40). New York: Random House.

Conrad, P. (1990). Qualitative research on chronic illness: A commentary on method and conceptual development. *Social Science & Medicine, 30*, 1257-1263.

Conrad, P., & Schneider, J. W. (1981). Professionalization, monopoly, and the structure of medical practice. In P. Conrad & R. Kern (Eds.), *The sociology of health and illness: Critical perspectives* (pp. 155-165). New York: St. Martin's.

Corbin, J. M., & Strauss, A. L. (1988). *Unending work and care: Managing chronic illness at home.* San Francisco: Jossey-Bass.

Crum, G. (1991). Professionalism and physician reimbursement. In J. D. Moreno (Ed.), *Paying the doctor: Health policy and physician reimbursement* (pp. 3-11). New York: Auburn House.

Curtin, M., & Lubkin, I. M. (1990). What is chronicity? In I. M. Lubkin (Ed.). *Chronic illness: Impact and interventions* (2nd ed., pp. 2-20). Boston: Jones & Bartlett.

Dallery, A. B. (1983). Illness and health: Alternatives to medicine. In W. L. McBride & C. O. Schrag (Eds.), *Phenomenology in a pluralistic society* (pp. 167-175). Albany: State University of New York Press.

Daniels, N. (1985). *Just health care.* Cambridge: Cambridge University Press.

Dean, K. (1986). Lay care in illness. *Social Science & Medicine, 22,* 275-284.

de Swaan, A. (1989). The reluctant imperialism of the medical profession. *Social Science & Medicine, 28,* 1165-1170.

de Vries, M. W., Berg, R. L., & Lipkin, M. (1982). On the use and abuse of medicine: A conclusion. In M. W. de Vries, R. L. Berg, & M. Lipkin (Eds.), *The use and abuse of medicine* (pp. 269-282). New York: Praeger.

DeVries, R. A. (1988). A balance: Cost, quality, and access. In W. K. Kellogg Foundation (Eds.), *Stemming the rising costs of medical care: Answers and antidotes* (pp. 219-222). Battle Creek, MI: W. K. Kellogg Foundation.

Diamond, M. (1983). Social adaptation of the chronically ill. In D. Mechanic (Ed.), *Handbook of health, health care, and the health professions* (pp. 636-654). New York: Free Press.

Drummond, M. F. (1987). Resource allocation decisions in health care: A role for quality of life assessments? *Journal of Chronic Diseases, 40,* 605-616.

Duff, R. S. (1988). Unshared and shared decision-making: Reflections on helplessness and healing. In N.M.P. King, L. R. Churchill, & A. W. Cross (Eds.), *The physician as captain of the ship: A critical appraisal* (pp. 191-221). Dordrecht, Holland: D. Reidel.

Duval, M. L. (1984). Psychosocial metaphors of physical distress among MS patients. *Social Science & Medicine, 19,* 635-638.

Evans, R. (1991). Health care in the 1990's: Universal issues, Canadian responses. In synopsis of conference proceedings: *Forum on health care: Where do we go from here?* (pp. 10-14). Victoria, BC: The Medical-Legal Society of British Columbia.

Fabrega, H. (1974). *Disease and social behavior: An interdisciplinary perspective.* Cambridge: MIT Press.

Fabrega, H. (1982). The idea of medicalization: An anthropological perspective. In M. W. de Vries, R. L. Berg, & M. Lipkin (Eds.), *The use and abuse of medicine* (pp. 19-35). New York: Praeger.

Ferguson, T. (1980). Medical self-care: Self-responsibility for health. In P.A.R. Flynn (Ed.), *The healing continuum: Journeys in the philosophy of holistic health* (pp. 391-408). Bowie, MD: Brady.

Fisher, S. (1984). Doctor-patient communication: A social and micro-political perfor-mance. *Sociology of Health & Illness, 6*(1), 1-29.

Fitzpatrick, R. M., Hopkins, A. P., & Harvard-Watts, O. (1983). Social dimensions of healing: A longitudinal study of outcomes of medical management of headaches. *Social Science & Medicine, 17,* 501-510.

Fox, R. C. (1986). Medicine, science, and technology. In L. H. Aiken & D. Mechanic (Eds.), *Applications of social science to clinical medicine and health policy* (pp. 13-30). New Brunswick, NJ: Rutgers University Press.

Fox, R. C. (1990). Training in caring competence in North American medicine. *Humane Medicine, 6*(1), 15-21.

Frankel, B. G., & Nutall, S. (1984). Illness behavior: An exploration of determinants. *Social Science & Medicine, 19*, 147-155.

Freel, M. (1985). Consumers' rights and the health care industry. In J. C. McCloskey & H. K. Grace (Eds.), *Current issues in nursing* (2nd ed., pp. 586-594). Boston: Blackwell Scientific Publications.

Freidson, E. (1981). Professional dominance and the ordering of health services: Some consequences. In P. Conrad & R. Kern (Eds.), *The sociology of health and illness* (pp. 184-197). New York: St. Martin's.

Freidson, E. (1986). The medical profession in transition. In L. H. Aiken & D. Mechanic (Eds.), *Application of social science to clinical medicine and health policy* (pp. 63-79). New Brunswick, NJ: Rutgers University Press.

Funkhouser, S. W., & Moser, D. K. (1990). Is health care racist? *Advances in Nursing Science, 12*(2), 47-55.

Gallagher, E. B. (1988). Chronic illness management: A focus for future research applications. In D. S. Gochman (Ed.), *Health behavior: Emerging research perspectives* (pp. 397-407). New York: Plenum.

Gerhardt, U. (1990). Qualitative research on chronic illness: The issue and the story. *Social Science & Medicine, 30*, 1149-1159.

Gething, L. (1992). Judgements by health professionals of personal characteristics of people with a visible physical disability. *Social Science & Medicine, 34*, 809-815.

Gilliss, C., Rose, D. B., Hallburg, J. C., & Martinson, I. M. (1989). The family and chronic illness. In C. L. Gilliss, B. L. Highley, B. M. Roberts, & I. Martinson (Eds.), *Toward a science of family nursing* (pp. 287-299). Menlo Park, CA: Addison-Wesley.

Gish, O. (1984). Values in health care. *Social Science & Medicine, 19*, 333-339.

Glaser, B. G., & Strauss, A. L. (1967). *The discovery of grounded theory: Strategies for qualitative research*. Chicago: Aldine.

Glaser, W. A. (1986). Payment systems and their effects. In L. H. Aiken & D. Mechanic (Eds.), *Applications of social science to clinical medicine and health policy* (pp. 481-499). New Brunswick, NJ: Rutgers University Press.

Griffith, B., Iliffe, S., & Rayner, G. (1987). *Banking on sickness: Commercial medicine in Britain and the USA*. London: Lawrence and Wishart.

Gubrium, J. (1988). *Analyzing field reality*. Newbury Park, CA: Sage.

Hahn, R. A., & Kleinman, A. (1983). Biomedical practice and anthropological theory. *Annual Review of Anthropology, 12*, 305-333.

Hahn, S. R., Feiner, J. S., & Bellin, E. H. (1988). The doctor-patient-family relationship: A compensatory alliance. *Annals of Internal Medicine, 109*, 884-889.

Halpern, K. G., Fisk, T. A., & Sobel, J. (1984). Consumer preference: The overlooked element in health planning. In J. M. Virgo (Ed.), *Health care: An international perspective* (pp. 267-278). Edwardsville, IL: International Health Economics and Management Institute.

Hancock, T. (1987). Healthy cities: The Canadian project. *Health Promotion, 26*(1), 2-4, 27.

Harris, J. S. (1989). What employers can do about medical care costs: Managing health and productivity. In K. McLennan & J. A. Meyer (Eds.), *Care and cost: Current issues in health policy* (pp. 167-202). Boulder, CO: Westview.

Hepburn, S. J. (1988). Western minds, foreign bodies. *Medical Anthropology Quarterly, 2*, 59-74.

Herzlich, C., & Graham, D. (1973). *Health and illness: A social psychological analysis.* London: Academic Press.

Herzlich, C., & Pierret, J. (1985). The social construction of the patient: Patients and illnesses in other ages. *Social Science Medicine, 20,* 145-151.

Hillier, S. (1987). Rationalism, bureaucracy, and the organization of the health services: Max Weber's contribution to understanding modern health care systems. In G. Scambler (Ed.), *Sociological theory and medical sociology* (pp. 194-220). London: Tavistock.

Hingson, R., Scotch, N. A., Sorenson, J., & Swazey, J. P. (1981). *In sickness and in health: Social dimensions of medical care.* St. Louis: Mosby.

Hunt, L. B. (1988). From a chain to a network: Trends and developments in the pattern of health care. In B.D.H. Doan (Ed.), *The future of health and health care systems in the industrialized world* (pp. 115-126). New York: Praeger.

Illich, I. (1975). *Medical nemesis: The expropriation of health.* London: Calder & Boyars.

Inlander, C. B., Levin, L. S., & Weiner, E. (1988). *Medicine on trial: The appalling story of medical ineptitude and the arrogance that overlooks it.* New York: Pantheon.

Jaspars, J., King, J., & Pendleton, D. (1983). The consultation: A social psychological analysis. In D. Pendleton & J. Hasler (Eds.), *Doctor-patient communication* (pp. 139-157). London: Academic Press.

Jekel, J. F. (1987). "Rainbow reviews" III: Recent publications of the National Center for Health Statistics. *Journal of Chronic Diseases, 40,* 439-443.

Kasl, S. V. (1983). Social and psychological factors affecting course of disease: An epidemiological perspective. In D. Mechanic (Ed.), *Handbook of health, health care, and the health professions* (pp. 683-708). New York: Free Press.

Katz, S. (1987). The science of quality of life. *Journal of Chronic Diseases, 40,* 459-463.

Kaufman, S. R. (1988). Toward a phenomenology of boundaries in medicine: Chronic illness experience in the case of stroke. *Medical Anthropology Quarterly, 2,* 338-354.

Kaufmann, C. (1987). Rights and the provision of health care: A comparison of Canada, Great Britain, and the United States. In H. D. Schwartz (Ed.), *Dominant issues in medical sociology* (pp. 491-510). New York: Random House.

Kleinman, A. (1980). *Patients and healers in the context of culture: An exploration of the borderland between anthropology, medicine and psychiatry.* Berkeley: University of California Press.

Kleinman, A. (1984). Indigenous systems of healing: Questions for professional, popular, and folk care. In J. W. Salmon (Ed.), *Alternative medicine: Popular and policy perspectives* (pp. 138-164). New York: Tavistock.

Kleinman, A., Eisenberg, L., & Good, B. (1978). Culture, illness and care: Clinical lessons from anthropologic and cross cultural research. *Annals of Internal Medicine, 88,* 251-258.

Knafl, K. A., & Deatrick, J. A. (1986). How families manage chronic conditions: An analysis of the concept of normalization. *Research in Nursing & Health, 9,* 215-222.

Knafl, K. A., & Webster, D. C. (1988). Managing and analyzing qualitative data: A description of tasks, techniques, and materials. *Western Journal of Nursing Research, 10,* 195-218.

Krefting, L. (1990). Double bind and disability: The case of traumatic head injury. *Social Science & Medicine, 30,* 859-865.

Labonte, R. (1987). Community health promotion strategies. *Health Promotion, 28*(1), 5-10, 32.

LaFargue, J. P. (1985). Mediating between two views of illness. *Topics in Clinical Nursing, 7*(3), 70-77.

LaLonde, M. (1980). The traditional view of the health field. In P.A.R. Flynn (Ed.), *The healing continuum: Journeys in the philosophy of holistic health* (pp. 439-464). Bowie, MD: Brady.

Lambert, C. E., & Lambert, V. A. (1987). Psychosocial impacts created by chronic illness. *Nursing Clinics of North America, 22,* 527-533.

Lambert, V. A., & Lambert, C. E. (1985). *Psychosocial care of the physically ill* (2nd ed.). Englewood Cliffs, NJ: Prentice-Hall.

Larkin, J. (1987). Factors influencing one's ability to adapt to chronic illness. *Nursing Clinics of North America, 22,* 535-542.

Last, J. M. (1987). *Public health and human ecology.* Norwalk, CT: Appleton & Lange.

Last, J. M. (1988). The future of health and health services. In B.D.H. Doan (Ed.), *The future of health and health care systems in the industrialized world* (pp. 20-34). New York: Praeger.

Lau, R. R., Williams, S., Williams, L. C., Ware, J. E., & Brook, R. H. (1982). Psychosocial problems in chronically ill children. *Journal of Community Health, 7*(4), 250-261.

Law, M., & Lariviere, J. (1988). Canada and WHO: Giving and receiving. *Health Promotion, 26*(4), 2-8, 16.

Lazarus, E. S., & Pappas, G. (1986). Categories of thought and critical theory: Anthropology and the social science of medicine. *Medical Anthropology Quarterly, 17,* 136-137.

Leahey, M., & Wright, L. M. (1987). Families and chronic illness: Assumptions, assessment, and intervention. In L. M. Wright & M. Leahey (Eds.), *Families and chronic illness* (pp. 55-76). Springhouse, PA: Springhouse Corporation.

Lenihan, S. (1981). Quest for meaning in the face of chronic illness. In B. J. Perdue, N. E. Mahon, S. L. Hawes, & S.M. Frik (Eds.), *Chronic care nursing* (pp. 33-38). New York: Springer.

Leventhal, H., Nerenz, D. R., & Straus, A. (1982). Self-regulation and the mechanisms for symptom appraisal. In D. Mechanic (Ed.), *Symptoms, illness behavior, and help-seeking* (pp. 55-86). New York: Prodist.

Levine, S., Feldman, J. J., & Elinson, J. (1983). Does medical care do any good? In D. Mechanic (Ed.), *Handbook of health, health care, and the health professions* (pp. 394-404). New York: Free Press.

Light, D. W. (1986). Surplus versus cost containment: The changing context for health providers. In L. H. Aiken & D. Mechanic (Eds.), *Applications of social science to clinical medicine and health policy* (pp. 519-542). New Brunswick, NJ: Rutgers University Press.

Like, R., & Zyanski, S. J. (1987). Patient satisfaction with the clinical encounter: Social psychological determinants. *Social Science & Medicine, 24,* 351-357.

Lincoln, Y. S., & Guba, E. G. (1985). *Naturalistic inquiry.* Beverly Hills: Sage.

Livneh, H. (1984). On the origins of negative attitudes toward people with disabilities. In R. P. Marinelli & A. E. Dell Orto (Eds.), *The psychological and social impact of physical disability* (pp. 167-184). New York: Springer.

Lohr, K. N., Kamberg, C. J., Keeler, E. B., Goldberg, G. A., Calabro, T. A., & Brook, R. H. (1987). Chronic disease in a general adult population: Findings from the Rand Health Insurance Experiment. *Connecticut Medicine, 51*(2), 87-96.

Lorber, J. (1979). Good patients and problem patients: Conformity and deviance in a general hospital. In E. G. Jaco (Ed.), *Patients, physicians, and illness* (pp. 202-217). New York: Free Press.

Lord, J. (1989). The potential of consumer participation: Sources of understanding. *Canada's Mental Health, 37*(2), 15-17.

Lubkin, I. M. (1990a). Chronic pain. In I. M. Lubkin (Ed.). *Chronic illness: Impact and interventions* (2nd ed., pp. 111-134). Boston: Jones & Bartlett.

Lubkin, I. M. (1990b). Illness roles. In I. M. Lubkin (Ed.). *Chronic illness: Impact and interventions* (2nd ed., pp. 43-64). Boston: Jones & Bartlett.

Luft, H. S. (1986). Economic incentives and constraints in clinical practice. In L. H. Aiken & D. Mechanic (Eds.), *Applications of social science to clinical medicine and health policy* (pp. 500-518). New Brunswick, NJ: Rutgers University Press.

Lynaugh, J. E. (1988). Narrow passageways: Nurses and physicians in conflict and concert since 1875. In N.M.P. King, L. R. Churchill, & A. W. Cross (Eds.), *The physician as captain of the ship: A critical reappraisal* (pp. 23-37). Boston: D. Reidel.

MacElveen-Hoehn, P. (1983). The cooperation model for care in health and illness. In N. L. Chaska (Ed.), *The nursing profession: A time to speak* (pp. 515-539). New York: McGraw-Hill.

MacGregor, J. (1974). Western beliefs and values and the quality of American life. In American Medical Association (Ed.), *Quality of life: The middle years* (pp. 19-26). Acton, MA: Publishing Sciences Group.

Mann, S. B. (1982). *Being ill: Personal and social meaning.* New York: Irvington.

Margolese, R. G. (1987). The place of psychosocial studies in medicine and surgery. *Journal of Chronic Diseases, 40*, 627-628.

Marmor, T. R., & Dunham, A. (1983). The politics of health. In D. Mechanic (Ed.), *Handbook of health, health care, and the health professions* (pp. 67-80). New York: Free Press.

Marshall, R. S. (1988). Interpretation in doctor-patient interviews: A sociolinguistic analysis. *Culture, Medicine & Psychiatry, 12*, 201-218.

McArt, E. W., & McDougal, L. W. (1985). Secondary data analysis: A new approach to nursing research. *Image: The Journal of Nursing Scholarship, 17*, 54-57.

McKee, J. (1988). Holistic health and the critique of western medicine. *Social Science & Medicine, 26*, 775-784.

McKeown, T. (1979). *The role of medicine.* Oxford: Blackwell.

McKeown, T. (1988). *The origins of human disease.* Oxford: Blackwell.

McKinlay, J. B. (1981a). A case for refocussing upstream: The political economy of illness. In P. Conrad & R. Kern (Eds.), *The sociology of health and illness: Critical perspectives* (pp. 613-633). New York: St. Martin's Press.

McKinlay, J. B. (1981b). Social network influences in morbid episodes and the career of help-seeking. In L. Eisenberg & A. Kleinman (Eds.), *The relevance of social science for medicine* (pp. 77-107). Boston: Reidel.

McKinlay, J. B., & McKinlay, S. M. (1987). Medical measures and the decline of mortality. In H. D. Schwartz (Ed.), *Dominant issues in medical sociology* (2nd ed., pp. 691-703). New York: Random House.

McKinlay, J. B., McKinlay, S. M., Jennings, S., & Grant, K. (1983). Mortality, morbidity, and the inverse care law. In A. L. Greer & S. Greer (Eds.), *Cities and sickness: Health care in urban America* (p. 99-138). Beverly Hills, CA: Sage.

McKinlay, J. B., & Stoeckle, J. D. (1988). Corporatization and the social transformation of doctoring. *International Journal of Health Services, 18*, 191-205.

McLennan, K., & Meyer, J. A. (1989). Containing health care cost escalation and improving access to services: The search for a solution. In K. McLennan & J. A. Meyer (Eds.), *Care and cost: Current issues in health policy* (pp. 1-11). Boulder, CO: Westview.

Mechanic, D. (1979a). *Future issues in health care: Social policy and the rationing of medical services.* New York: Free Press.

Mechanic, D. (1979b). The growth of medical technology and bureaucracy: Implications for medical care. In E. G. Jaco (Ed.), *Patients, physicians, and illness* (pp. 405-417). New York: Free Press.

Mechanic, D. (1983). The experience and expression of distress: The study of illness behavior and medical utilization. In D. Mechanic (Ed.), *Handbook of health, health care, and the health professions* (pp. 591-607). New York: Free Press.

Mechanic, D. (1986a). *From advocacy to allocation: The evolving American health care system.* New York: Free Press.

Mechanic, D. (1986b). The concept of illness behavior: Culture, situation and personal disposition. *Psychological Medicine, 16,* 1-7.

Mechanic, D. (1987). A brief anatomy of the American health care system. In H. D. Schwartz (Ed.), *Dominant issues in medical sociology* (2nd ed., pp. 462-475). New York: Random House.

Mechanic, D. (1989). *Painful choices: Research and essays on health care.* New Brunswick, NJ: Transaction Books.

Mechanic, D., & Aiken, L. H. (1986). Social science, medicine, and health policy. In L. H. Aiken & D. Mechanic (Eds.), *Applications of social science to clinical medicine and health policy* (pp. 1-9). New Brunswick, NJ: Rutgers University Press.

Meister, S. B. (1989). Health care financing, policy and family nursing practice. In C. L. Gilliss, B. L. Highly, B. M. Roberts, & I. Martinson (Eds.), *Toward a science of family nursing.* Menlo Park, CA: Addison-Wesley.

Meleis, A. I. (1988). The sick role. In M. E. Hardy & M. E. Conway (Eds.), *Role theory: Perspectives for health professionals* (2nd ed., pp. 365-374). Norwalk, CT: Appleton & Lange.

Meyerson, A. T., & Herman, G. H. (1987). Systems resistance to the chronic patient. In A. T. Meyerson (Ed.), *Barriers to treating the chronically mentally ill* (pp. 21-33). San Francisco: Jossey-Bass.

Mikhail, B. (1981). The health belief model: A review and critical evaluation of the model, research, and practice. *Advances in Nursing Science, 4*(1), 65-82.

Milio, N. (1988). Public policy as the cornerstone for a new public health: Local and global beginnings. *Family and Community Health, 11*(2), 57-71.

Mishler, E. G. (1981). The social construction of illness. In E. G. Mishler, L. Amara-Singham, S. Hauser, R. Liem, S. Osherson, & N. E. Waxler (Eds.), *Social contexts of health, illness and patient care* (pp. 141-168). Cambridge: Cambridge University Press.

Mishler, E. G. (1984). *The discourse of medicine: Dialectics of medical interviews.* Norwood, NJ: Ablex.

Mizrahi, T. (1986). *Getting rid of patients: Contradictions in the socialization of physicians.* New Brunswick, NJ: Rutgers University Press.

Moos, R. H., & Tsu, V. D. (1977). The crisis of physical illness: An overview. In R. H. Moos (Ed.), *Coping with physical illness* (pp. 3-21). New York: Plenum.

Morgan, M., Calnan, M., & Manning, N. (1985). *Sociological approaches to health and medicine.* London: Croom Helm.

Morse, J. M., & Johnson, J. L. (1991). Toward a theory of illness: The illness constellation model. In J. M. Morse & J. L. Johnson (Eds.), *The illness experience: Dimensions of suffering* (pp. 315-342). Beverly Hills, CA: Sage.

Murphy, R. F., Scheer, J., Murphy, Y., & Mack, R. (1988). Physical disability and social liminality: A study in the rituals of adversity. *Social Science & Medicine, 26,* 235-242.

Myers, G. C. (1988). Chronic non-life-threatening health ailments: An overlooked dimension. In B.D.H. Doan (Ed.), *The future of health and health care systems in the industrialized societies* (pp. 67-80). New York: Praeger.

Navarro, V. (1984). Selected myths guiding the Reagan administration's health policies. *International Journal of Health Services, 14,* 321-328.

Navarro, V. (1986). *Crisis, health, and medicine: A social critique.* New York: Tavistock.

Navarro, V. (1989). Why some countries have national health insurance, others have national health services, and the U.S. has neither. *Social Science & Medicine, 28,* 887-898.

Nield, L. J., & Mahon, N. E. (1981). Barriers to health care. In B. J. Perdue, N. E. Mahon, S. L. Hawes, & S. M. Frik (Eds.), *Chronic care nursing* (pp. 26-32). New York: Springer.

Nordstrom, M., & Lubkin, I. M. (1990). Quality of life. In I. M. Lubkin (Ed.), *Chronic illness: Impact and interventions* (2nd ed., pp. 136-154). Boston: Jones & Bartlett.

O'Neill, J. (1985). *Five bodies: The human shape of modern society.* Ithaca, NY: Cornell University Press.

O'Neill, J. (1986). The medicalization of social control. *Canadian Review of Sociology and Anthropology, 23,* 350-364.

O'Neill, M. (1989/90). Healthy public policy: The WHO perspective. *Health Promotion, 28*(3), 6-8, 24.

Paget, M. A. (1983). On the work of talk: Studies in misunderstanding. In S. Fisher & A. D. Todd (Eds.), *The social organization of doctor-patient communication* (pp. 55-74). Washington, DC: Center for Applied Linguistics.

Parsons, T. (1951). *The social system.* New York: Free Press.

Parsons, T. (1979). Definitions of health and illness in the light of American values and social structure. In E. G. Jaco (Ed.), *Patients, physicians, and illness* (pp. 120-144). New York: Free Press.

Pellegrino, E. D. (1982). Being ill and being healed: Some reflections on the grounding of medical morality. In V. Kestenbaum (Ed.), *The humanity of the ill: Phenomenological perspectives* (pp. 157-166). Knoxville: University of Tennessee Press.

Pellegrino, E. D., & Thomasma, D. C. (1988). *For the patient's good: The restoration of beneficence in health care.* New York: Oxford University Press.

Pelletier, K. (1980). Toward a holistic medicine. In P.A.R. Flynn (Ed.), *The healing continuum: Journeys in the philosophy of holistic health* (pp. 419-434). Bowie, MD: Brady.

Pelto, P. J., & DeWalt, B. R. (1985). Methodology in macro-micro studies. In B. R. DeWalt & P. J. Pelto (Eds.), *Micro and macro levels of analysis in anthropology: Issues in theory and research* (pp. 187-201). Boulder, CO: Westview.

Pendleton, D. (1983). Doctor-patient communication: A review. In D. Pendleton & J. Halser (Eds.), *Doctor-patient communication* (pp. 5-53). London: Academic Press.

Phillips, M. J. (1990). Damaged goods: Oral narratives of the experience of disability in American culture. *Social Science & Medicine, 30,* 849-857.

Preston, T. A. (1986). *The clay pedestal* (rev. ed.). New York: Scribner.

Pritchard, P. (1983). Patient participation. In D. Pendleton & J. Hasler (Eds.), *Doctor-patient communication* (pp. 205-223). London: Academic Press.

Rabin, D., & Rabin, P. L. (1985). The pariah syndrome: The social disease of chronic illness. In P. L. Rabin & D. Rabin (Eds.), *To provide safe passage: The humanistic aspects of medicine* (pp. 38-47). New York: Philosophical Library.

Rabin, D., Rabin, P. L., & Rabin, R. C. (1985). Compounding the ordeal of ALS: Isolation from my fellow physicians. In P. L. Rabin & D. Rabin (Eds.), *To provide safe passage: The humanistic aspects of medicine* (pp. 29-37). New York: Philosophical Library.

Rachlis, M. (1991). Strategic planning for health: What can be learned from the other provinces. In synopsis of conference proceedings: *Forum on health care: Where do we go from here?* (pp. 15-19). Victoria, BC: The Medical-Legal Society of British Columbia.

Rachlis, M., & Kushner, C. (1989). *Second opinion: What's wrong with Canada's health care system and how to fix it.* Toronto: Harper & Collins.

Radley, A. (1989). Style, discourse and constraint in adjustment to chronic illness. *Sociology of Health & Illness, 11,* 230-252.

Rawlinson, M. C. (1983). The facticity of illness and the appropriation of health. In W. L. McBride & C. O. Schwag (Eds.), *Phenomenology in a pluralistic context* (pp. 155-166). Albany: State University of New York Press.

Relman, A. S. (1987). The new medical-industrial complex. In H. D. Schwartz (Ed.), *Dominant issues in medical sociology* (2nd ed., pp. 597-608). New York: Random House.

Roberson, M.H.B. (1987). Folk health beliefs of health professionals. *Western Journal of Nursing Research, 9,* 257-263.

Robinson, C. A., & Thorne, S. E. (1985). Strengthening family "interference." *Journal of Advanced Nursing, 9,* 597-602.

Robinson, E. J., & Whitfield. (1988). Contributions of patients to general practitioner consultations in relation to their understanding of doctor's instructions and advice. *Social Science & Medicine, 27,* 895-900.

Rogers, W. R., & Barnard, D. (1979). Some policy implications and recommendations. In W. R. Rogers & D. Barnard (Eds.), *Nourishing the humanistic in medicine: Interactions with the social sciences* (pp. 297-305). Pittsburgh: University of Pittsburgh Press.

Rolland, J. S. (1987). Chronic illness and the family: An overview. In L. M. Wright & M. Leahey (Eds.), *Families & chronic illness* (pp. 33-54). Springhouse, PA: Springhouse Corporation.

Rolland, J. S. (1988). A conceptual model of chronic and life-threatening illness and its impact on families. In C. S. Chilman, E. W. Nunnally, & F. M. Fox (Eds.), *Chronic illness and disability* (pp. 17-68). Newbury Park, CA: Sage.

Romanucci-Ross, L. (1982). Folk medicine and metaphor in the context of medicalization: Syncretics in curing practices. In L. Romanucci-Ross, D. E. Moerman, & L. R. Tancredi (Eds.), *The anthropology of medicine: From culture to method* (pp. 5-19). New York: Praeger.

Rosenstein, A. H. (1986). Consumerism and health care: Will the traditional patient-physician relationship survive? *Postgraduate Medicine, 79,* 13-18.

Rosenstock, I. M. (1966). Why people use health services. *Millbank Memorial Fund Quarterly, 44,* 97-127.

Ruffing-Rahal, M. A. (1985). Well-being and chronicity: Being singular rather than sick. *Health Values, 9*(5), 17-22.

Salmon, J. W. (1984). Defining health and reorganizing medicine. In J. W. Salmon (Ed.), *Alternative medicine: Popular and policy perspectives* (pp. 252-288). New York: Tavistock.

Salmond, S. W. (1987). Health care needs of the chronically ill. *Orthopedic Nursing, 6*(6), 39-45.

Sandelowski, M. (1986). The problem of rigor in qualitative research. *Advances in Nursing Science, 8*(3), 27-37.

Sanders, D. (1985). *The struggle for health: Medicine and the politics of underdevelopment.* London: Macmillan.

Scambler, G. (1984). Perceiving and coping with stigmatizing illness. In R. Fitzpatrick, J. Hinton, S. Newman, G. Scambler, & J. Thompson (Eds.), *The experience of illness* (pp. 201-226). London: Tavistock.

Scambler, G., & Hopkins, A. (1986). Being epileptic: Coming to terms with stigma. *Sociology of Health & Illness, 8*, 26-43.

Scheff, T. J. (1986). Toward resolving the controversy over "thick description." *Current Anthropology, 27*, 408-409.

Schilling, J. (1981). Ethical issues related to chronic disease. In S. V. Anderson & E. E. Bauwens (Eds.), *Chronic health problems: Concepts and application* (pp. 291-304). St. Louis: Mosby.

Schlesinger, M. (1986). On the limits of expanding health care reform: Chronic care in prepaid settings. *Millbank Memorial Fund Quarterly, 64*, 189-215.

Schwartz, H. D. (1987). Irrationality as a feature of health care in the United States. In H. D. Schwartz (Ed.), *Dominant issues in medical sociology* (2nd ed., pp. 475-490). New York: Random House.

Sherlock, R. (1986). Reasonable men and sick human beings. *The American Journal of Medicine, 80*, 2-4.

Shonz, F. C. (1984). Psychological adjustment to physical disability: Trends in theories. In R. P. Marinelli & A. E. Dell Orto (Eds.), *The psychological and social impact of physical disability* (pp. 119-126). New York: Springer.

Shorter, E. (1985). *Bedside manners: The troubled history of doctors and patients.* New York: Simon & Schuster.

Siler-Wells, G. (1988). Public participation in community health. *Health Promotion, 27*(1), 7-11, 23.

Simmons, R. G., & Marine, S. K. (1984). The regulation of high cost technology medicine: The case of dialysis and transplantation in the United Kingdom. *Journal of Health and Social Behavior, 25*, 320-334.

Sparr, L. F., Gordon, G. H., Hickam, D. H., & Girard, D. E. (1988). The doctor-patient relationship during medical internship: The evolution of dissatisfaction. *Social Science & Medicine, 26*, 1095-1101.

Spicker, S. F. (1988). Marketing health care: Ethical challenge to physicians. In N.M.P. King, L. R. Churchill, & A. W. Cross (Eds.), *The physician as captain of the ship: A critical reappraisal* (pp. 159-176). Boston: D. Reidel.

Starr, P. (1981). The politics of therapeutic nihilism. In P. Conrad & R. Kern (Eds.), *The sociology of health and illness* (pp. 434-448). New York: St. Martin's.

Stephenson, J. S., & Murphy, D. (1986). Existential grief: The special case of the chronically ill and disabled. *Death Studies, 10*, 133-145.

Strauss, A. (1981). Chronic illness. In P. Conrad & R. Kern (Eds.), *The sociology of health and illness: Critical perspectives* (pp. 138-149). New York: St. Martin's.

Strauss, A. (1990). A trajectory model for reorganizing the health care system. In *Perspectives in Nursing 1989-1991* (pp. 221-231). New York: National League for Nursing.

Strauss, A., & Corbin, J. M. (1988). *Shaping a new health care system: The explosion of chronic illness as a catalyst for change.* San Francisco: Jossey-Bass.

Strauss, A., & Corbin, J. (1990). *Basics of qualitative research: Grounded theory procedures and techniques.* Newbury Park, CA: Sage.

Strauss, A. L., Corbin, J., Fagerhaugh, S., Glaser, B. G., Maines, D., Suczek, B., & Wiener, C. L. (1984). *Chronic illness and the quality of life* (2nd ed.). St. Louis: Mosby.

Strauss, A. L., Fagerhaugh, S., Suczek, B., & Weiner, C. (1981). Patient work in the technological hospital. *Nursing Outlook, 29*, 404-412.

Sullivan, M. (1986). In what sense is contemporary medicine dualistic? *Culture, Medicine & Psychiatry, 10*, 331-350.

Sullivan, P. (1990). The AMA looks north with fear and loathing. *Canadian Medical Association Journal, 142*, 50-51.

Susser, M., Hopper, K., & Richman, J. (1983). Society, culture, and health. In D. Mechanic (Ed.), *Handbook of health, health care, and the health professions* (pp. 23-49). New York: Free Press.

Swartz, D. (1977). The politics of reform: Conflict and accommodation in Canadian health policy. In L. Panitch (Ed.), *The Canadian state: Political economy and political power* (p. 311-343). Toronto: University of Toronto Press.

Szasz, T., & Hollender, M. (1980). A contribution to the philosophy of medicine: The basic models of the doctor-patient relationship. In P.A.R. Flynn (Ed.), *The healing continuum: Journeys in the philosophy of holistic health* (pp. 307-318). Bowie, MD: Brady. (Original work published 1956)

Tagliacozzo, D. L., & Mauksch, H. O. (1979). Caring for the ill: The patient role. In E. G. Jaco (Ed.), *Patients, physicians, and illness* (pp. 185-201). New York: Free Press.

Taylor, C. (1970). *Horizontal orbit: Hospitals and the cult of efficiency.* New York: Holt, Rinehart & Winston.

Taylor, R. (1979). *Medicine out of control: The anatomy of a malignant technology.* Melbourne: Sun Books.

Taylor, R.C.R. (1984). Alternative medicine and the medical encounter in Britain and the United States. In J. W. Salmon (Ed.), *Alternative medicines: Popular and policy perspectives* (pp. 191-228). New York: Tavistock.

Thomas, R. B. (1987). Family adaptation to a child with a chronic condition. In M. H. Rose & R. B. Thomas (Eds.), *Children with chronic conditions: Nursing in a family and community context* (pp. 29-54). Orlando, FL: Grune & Stratton.

Thomasma, D. C. (1984). The goals of medicine and society. In D. H. Brock & A. Harward (Eds.), *The culture of biomedicine: Studies in science and culture* (pp. 34-54). Newark: University of Delaware Press.

Thorne, S. E. (1985). The family cancer experience. *Cancer Nursing, 8*, 285-291.

Thorne, S. E. (1986). Life after cancer: The transition to wellness. *Nursing Research: Science for Quality Care, Proceedings of the Tenth National Research Conference* (pp. 118-121), Toronto.

Thorne, S. E. (1988). Helpful and unhelpful communications in cancer care: The patient perspective. *Oncology Nursing Forum, 15*, 167-172.

Thorne, S. E. (1990a). Constructive non-compliance in chronic illness. *Holistic Nursing Practice, 5*(1), 62-69.

Thorne, S. E. (1990b). Mothers with chronic illness: A predicament of social construction. *Health Care for Women International, 11*, 209-221.

Thorne, S. E., & Robinson, C. A. (1988a). Health care relationships: The chronic illness perspective. *Research in Nursing & Health, 11*, 293-300.

Thorne, S. E., & Robinson, C. A. (1988b). Legacy of the country doctor. *Journal of Gerontological Nursing, 14*(5), 23-26.

Thorne, S. E., & Robinson, C. A. (1988c). Reciprocal trust in health care relationships. *Journal of Advanced Nursing, 13*, 782-789.

Thorne, S. E., & Robinson, C. A. (1989). Guarded alliance: Health care relationships in chronic illness. *Image: The Journal of Nursing Scholarship, 21*, 153-157.

Tilden, V. P., & Weinert, C. (1987). Social support and the chronically ill individual. *Nursing Clinics of North America, 22*, 613-620.

Todd, A.D.T. (1989). *Intimate adversaries: Cultural conflict between doctors and women patients*. Philadelphia: University of Pennsylvania Press.

Tomes, N. (1985). The social transformation of American medicine: An historical perspective. *Sociology of Health & Illness, 7*, 248-254.

Travis, J. W. (1980). Wellness education: A new model for health care. In P.A.R. Flynn (Ed.), *The healing continuum: Journeys in the philosophy of holistic health* (pp. 339-352). Bowie, MD: Brady.

Turner, J. H. (1986). *The structure of sociological theory* (4th ed.). Chicago: Dorsey.

van der Steen, W. J., & Thung, P. J. (1988). *Faces of medicine: A philosophical study*. Dordrecht, Holland: Kluwer.

Viney, L. L. (1983). *Images of illness*. Malabar, FL: R. E. Krieger.

Vojtecky, M. A. (1986). A unified approach to health promotion and health protection. *Journal of Community Health, 11*, 219-221.

Waitzkin, H. (1983a). A Marxist view of health and health care. In D. Mechanic (Ed.), *Handbook of health, health care, and the health professions* (pp. 657-682). New York: Free Press.

Waitzkin, H. (1983b). *The second sickness: Contradictions of capitalist heath care*. New York: Free Press.

Waitzkin, H. (1984). The micropolitics of medicine: A contextual analysis. *International Journal of Health Services, 14*, 339-378.

Waitzkin, H. (1986). Micropolitics of medicine: Theoretical issues. *Medical Anthropology Quarterly, 17*, 134-136.

Walkover, M. (1988). Social policies: Understanding their impact on families with impaired members. In C. S. Chilman, E. W. Nunnally, & F. M. Cox (Eds.), *Chronic illness and disability* (pp. 220-247). Newbury Park, CA: Sage.

Warr, W. (1981). Toward a higher level of wellness: Prevention of chronic disease. In S. V. Anderson & E. E. Bauwens (Eds.), *Chronic health problems: Concepts and application* (pp. 18-29). St. Louis: Mosby.

Watts, R. J. (1990). Democratization of health care: Challenge for nursing. *Advances in Nursing Science, 12*(2), 37-46.

West, C. (1984). When the doctor is a "lady": Power, status and gender in physician-patient encounters. *Symbolic Interaction, 7*(1), 87-106.

Wiener, C., Fagerhaugh, S., Strauss, A., & Suczek, B. (1984). What price chronic illness? In A. L. Strauss (Ed.), *Where medicine fails* (4th ed., pp. 13-36). New Brunswick, NJ: Transaction Books.

Williams, G. H. (1989). Hope for the humblest? The role of self-help in chronic illness: The case of ankylosing spondylitis. *Sociology of Health & Illness, 11*, 135-159.

Williams, G. H. (1991). Disablement and the ideological crisis in health care. *Social Science & Medicine, 32*, 517-524.

Wolfensberger, W. (1980a). A brief overview of the principle of normalization. In R. J. Flynn & K. E. Nitsch (Eds.), *Normalization, social integration, and community services* (pp. 7-30). Baltimore: University Park Press.

Wolfensberger, W. (1980b). The definition of normalization: Update, problems, disagreements, and misunderstandings. In R. J. Flynn & K. E. Nitsch (Eds.), *Normalization, social integration, and community services* (pp. 71-115). Baltimore: University Park Press.

Wood-Dauphinee, S., & Williams, J.I. (1987). Reintegration to normal living as a proxy to quality of life. *Journal of Chronic Diseases, 40*, 491-499.

Woods, N. F. (1988). Using existing data sources: Primary and secondary analysis. In N. F. Woods & M. Catanzaro, *Nursing research: Theory and practice* (pp. 334-347). St. Louis: Mosby.

Woods, N. F., Yates, B. C., & Primomo, J. (1989). Supporting families during chronic illness. *Image: The Journal of Nursing Scholarship, 21*(1), 46-50.

Worsley, P. (1982). Non-western medical systems. *Annual Review of Anthropology, 11*, 315-348.

Wright, W. (1982). *The social logic of health*. New Brunswick, NJ: Rutgers University Press.

Yoder, L., & Jones, S. L. (1982). The family of the emergency room patient as seen through the eyes of the nurse. *International Journal of Nursing Studies, 19*(1), 29-36.

Young, A. (1982). The anthropologies of illness and sickness. *Annual Review of Anthropology, 11*, 257-285.

Zaner, R. M. (1983). Flirtations or engagements?: Prolegomenon to a philosophy of medicine. In W. L. McBride & C. O. Schrag (Eds.), *Phenomenology in a pluralistic society* (pp. 139-154). Albany: State University of New York Press.

Zaner, R. M. (1984). The phenomenon of medicine: Of hoaxes and humor. In D. H. Brock & A. Harwood (Eds.), *The culture of biomedicine*. Newark: University of Delaware Press.

Zola, I. K. (1973). Pathways to the doctor: From person to patient. *Social Science & Medicine, 7*, 677-689.

Zola, I. K. (1981). Medicine as an institution of social control. In P. Conrad & R. Kern (Eds.), *The sociology of health and illness: Critical perspectives* (pp. 511-527). New York: St. Martin's Press.

Zola, I. K. (1982). *Missing pieces: A chronicle of living with a disability*. Philadelphia: Temple University Press.

Author Index

Subject Index

About the Author

Sally E. Thorne, R.N., Ph.D., is an Associate Professor of Nursing at the University of British Columbia. She brings to this work 20 years of experience working with chronically ill patients as a clinician, an educator, and a researcher. Further, her active involvement with various community-based health care and social policy organizations over this period of time has helped her appreciate the imperative of understanding the links between the theoretical and the practical, the pure and the applied, the ideals within health care and the realities as they exist in the lives of those who experience illness in our society.

Dr. Thorne was born in the United Kingdom in 1951, and spent her formative years in Canada and India. She became a registered nurse in 1972. Interspersing periods of clinical practice with periods of study, she obtained her B.S.N. in 1979, her M.S.N. in 1983 (both from the University of British Columbia) and her Ph.D. (Nursing and Anthropology) in 1990 (from Union Institute in Cincinnati, Ohio). She has been a full-time faculty member at the University of British Columbia School of Nursing since 1983.